Legal Notice:

Disclaimer Notice:

TABLE OF CONTENTS

Introduction

Although ketogenic diet has been around for almost a century, it is rapidly gaining popularity today. There is a reason why keto is so highly regarded. It's not a fad diet. It actually works, and it has tremendous health benefits in addition to weight loss. When on the keto diet, you are feeding your body exactly what it needs, while eliminating toxins that will slow it down.

The keto diet focuses on low carbohydrates, which the body converts into energy to help speed up weight loss.

What exactly is the problem with high carbs, and why should you avoid them? Carbohydrates are converted into glucose and cause a spike in insulin. As the insulin enters the bloodstream to process the glucose, which becomes the main source of energy. A spike in insulin can also result in storage of fats. The body uses carbohydrates and fats as energy, the former being the primary source. So the more carbs you consume in your daily diet, the less fat is being burned for energy. Instead, the spike in insulin will result in more fat storage.

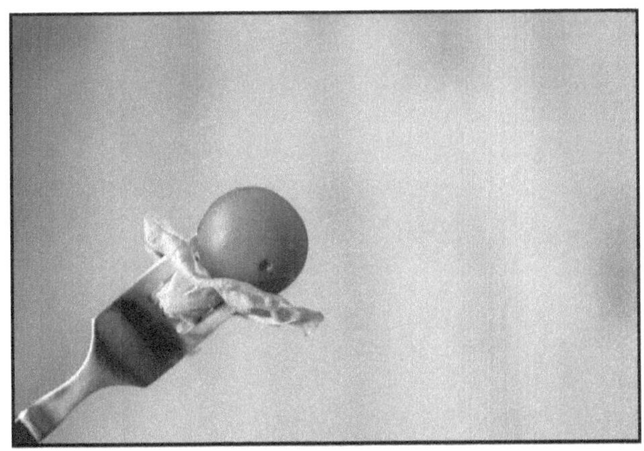

When you consume less carbohydrates, the body goes into a state referred to as ketosis. Thus, the name for this low-carb diet.

Ketosis helps the body survive on less food. By being in ketosis, you 'train' your Body to utilize fats as the main source of energy instead of carbs, simply because there is close to zero carbs to begin with. During ketosis, the liver breaks down fats into ketones, which enables the body to use the fat as energy. During a keto diet, we don't starve ourselves of calories; we starve the Body of carbohydrates. This makes weight loss easy and natural. Later on,
you'll learn that the keto diet has many additional health benefits besides fat loss.

The keto diet is an easy diet, but some people do miss beans and breads. It takes a bit of getting used to, starting anything new is challenging after all. But ultimately, you'll feel much better, both physically and mentally that you'd be happy to avoid carbs once and for all. And being able to eat bacon on a diet does have its rewards!

WHAT IS
KETOGENIC DIET?

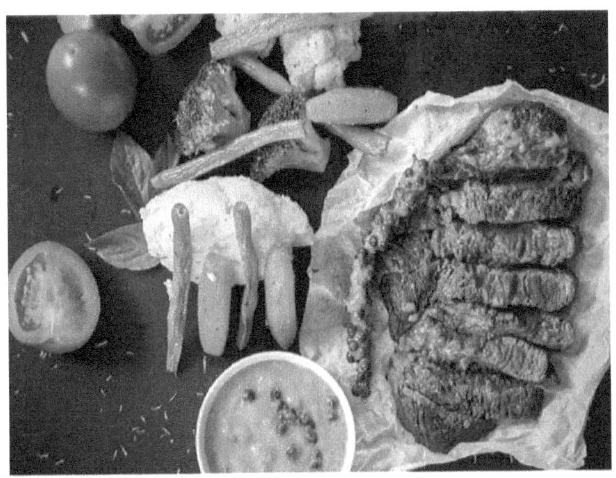

What is Ketogenic Diet?

The keto diet is a low or zero carbohydrate diet, but it differs from other low-carb diets (such as Paleo) in that it deliberately manipulates the ratios of carbs, fats, and protein to switch fat into the body's primary source of fuel. Our bodies are used to using carbohydrates as fuel. Fats, which is a secondary source of fuel, are rarely tapped on. That means the extra fat is stored and keeps adding on the pounds.
The only ways to reduce fat in a 'normal' diet are to consume less fat and workout a lot in order to increase energy expenditure over daily calories intake, which is why most people fail to lose weight on conventional diet.

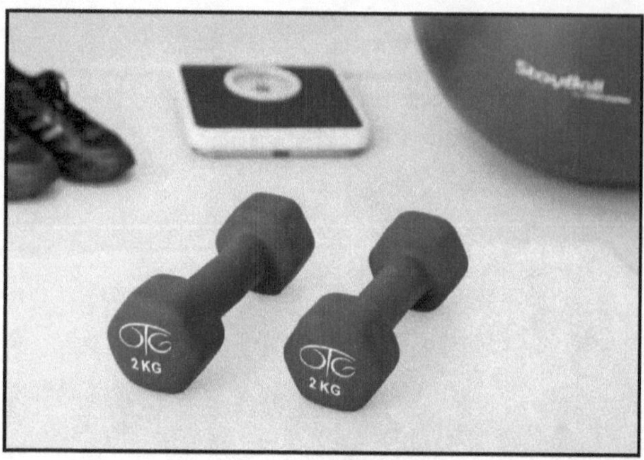

On the other hand, the ketogenic diet uses fat for fuel, which means it gets used instead of being stored. So, weight loss becomes easy. In addition to weight loss, the ketogenic diet is known as the "healing" diet. The lack of sugar intake has been proven to help and prevent many diseases such as heart disease, high blood pressure, cancers, epilepsy, and many symptoms of aging.

The manipulation of carbs, fats, and protein is curcial in order to get into ketosis. It's a state when the body, deprived of the usual carbohydrates and sugar, is forced to use fat as its primary fuel. So the ratio of fats and protein are significantly higher than carbs in general.

Of course, consuming less carbs also means lowering the amount of insulin in your body. Less insulin; Less glucose and fat storage. That is why the keto diet has been so successful in helping people with diabetes. It adjusts the sugar level naturally.

The ratio of carbs, fat, and protein can vary. Many people allow themselves up to 50 grams of carbohydrates a day and still lose weight. On a stricter regime, the carb intake can be between 15 and 20 grams daily. The less carbs, the quicker the weight loss, but the diet is very flexible.

On the keto diet, you don't count calories. You count carbohydrates and adjust the intake of carbs vs. fat and protein. A typical keto diet will get 60 percent of its calories from fat, 15 to 25 percent of calories from protein, and 25 percent of calories from carbohydrates. The only limitation on the diet is sugar, which you need to avoid.

The ketogenic diet is not a fad. Many scientific studies have shown the benefits and healing effects of ketosis. Discuss the ketogenic diet with your doctor if you are interested in consuming less sugar losing weight, or as preventive measures against vulnerable health problems.

BENEFITS OF KETO DIET

Benefits of Keto Diet

Although ketogenic diet is popularly known as a 'rapid fat loss diet', it is actually more to this than meets the eye. In fact, weight loss and higher levels of energy are only by-products of the keto diet, a kind of bonus. It has been scientifically proven that the keto diet has many additional medical benefits.

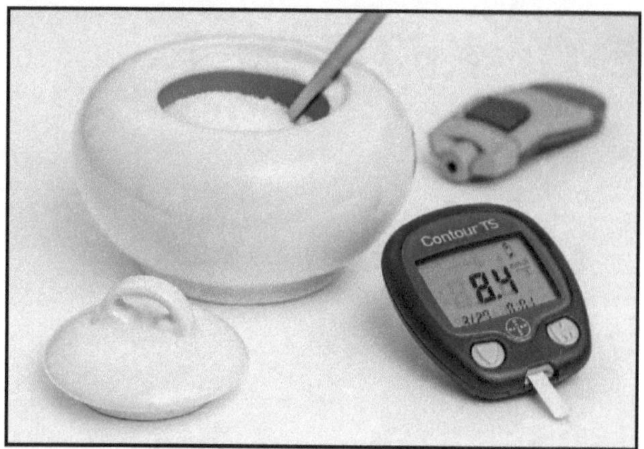

Let's begin by stating that a high carbohydrate diet, with its many processed ingredients and sugars, has absolutely no health benefits. These are merely empty calories, and most processed foods ultimately serve only to rob your body of the nutrients it needs to remain healthy. Here is a list of actual benefits for lowering your carbohydrates and eating fats that convert to energy:

Control of Blood Sugar

Keeping blood sugar at a low level is critical to manage and prevent diabetes. The keto diet has been proven to be extremely effective in preventing diabetes.
Many people suffering from diabetes are also overweight. That makes an easy weight-loss regime a natural. But the keto diet does more. Carbohydrates get converted to sugar, which for diabetics can result in a sugar spike. A diet low in carbohydrates prevents these spikes and allows more control over blood sugar levels.

Mental Focus

The keto diet is based on protein, fats, and low carbohydrates. As we've discussed, this forces fat to become the primary source of energy. This is not the normal western diet, which can be quite

deficient in nutrients, particularly fatty acids, which are needed for proper brain function.

When people suffer from cognitive diseases, such as Alzheimer's, the brain isn't using enough glucose, thus becomes lacking in energy, and the brain has difficulty functioning at a high level. The keto diet provides an additional energy source for the brain.

A study by the American Diabetes Association found that Type 1 diabetics improved their brain function after consuming coconut-oil.

That same study indicated that people who suffer from Alzheimer's may experience improved memory capacity on a keto diet. Those with Alzheimer's have seen improved memory scores that might correlate with the amount of ketones levels present.

What does this study mean to an average person? With the emphasis on fatty acids, such as omega 3 and omega 6 found in seafood, the keto diet is likely to fuel the brain with the additional nutrients to help achieve a healthier mental state. The brain tissue is made up largely of fatty acids (you've heard fish referred to as "brainfood"), and the increased consumption of those fatty acids will logically lead to improved brain health.

Our body does not produce fatty acids on its own; we can only obtain it through our diet. And the keto diet is rich in fatty acids.

A diet high in carbohydrates can lead to a "foggy" brain, where you have difficulty in focusing. Focusing becomes easier with the increased energy provided by the keto diet. In fact, many people who have no need or desire to lose weight use the keto diet to improve and enhance brain functions.

Increased Energy

It's not unusual, and has become almost normal, to feel tired and drained at the end of the day as a result of a poor, carbohydrate-laden diet. Fat is a more efficient source of energy, leaving you feeling more vitalized than you would on a "sugar" rush.

Acne

While most of the benefits of a keto diet are well-documented, one benefit catches some people by surprise: better skin and less acne. Acne is fairly common. Ninety percent of teens suffer from it, and many adults do, as well.

While it was always thought that acne was at least exacerbated by poor diet, controlled research is still being conducted. However, many people on the keto diet have reported clearer skin. There may be a logical reason. A 1972 study found that high levels of insulin can cause the eruption of acne. Since a keto diet keeps insulin at a low and healthy level, it may very well affect skin health.

In addition, acne thrives on inflammation. The ketogenic diet eases and reduces inflammation, thus enabling the body to decrease acne eruptions. Fatty acids, which are found in abundance in fish, are a known anti-inflammatory.

While research is still being done, it seems likely that a keto diet has beneficial effects for clearer, healthier, more glowing skin.

Keto and Anti-Aging

Many diseases are a natural result of the aging process. While there have not been studies done on humans, studies on mice have shown brain cell improvement on a keto diet.

Several studies have shown a positive effect of the keto diet on patients with Alzheimer's disease. What we do know is that a diet filled with good nutrients and antioxidants, low in sugar, high in protein and healthy fats, while low in carbohydrates, enhances our overall health. It protects us from the toxins of a poor diet.
There is also research indicating that using fatty acids for fuel instead of sugar may slow down the aging process, possibly because of the negative effects that sugar has on our overall wellbeing.
In addition, the simple act of eating less and consuming fewer calories is a matter of basic health, as it prevents obesity and its inherent side effects.
So far, studies have been limited. However, considering the powerful positive effects

of the ketogenic diet on our health, it is logical to assume this diet will help us grow older in a more natural way while delaying the natural effect of aging. A normal western diet laden with sugars and processed foods are certainly detrimental to warding off the signs of aging.

Keto and Hunger

One of the major reasons diets fail is hunger. People who diet feel hungry and deprived and simply give up. A low carbohydrate diet naturally leaves people feeling full and satisfied. Less hungry means people will actually remain on the diet longer while consuming fewer calories.

Keto and Eyesight

Diabetics are aware that high blood sugar can lead to a higher risk of developing cataracts. Since the keto diet controls sugar levels, it can help retain eyesight and help prevent cataracts. This has been proven in several studies involving diabetic patients.

Keto and Autism

We know the keto diet affects brain functions. In a study on autism, it was found that it also has a positive effect on autism. Thirty autistic children were placed on the keto diet. All showed improved in autistic behavior, especially those on the milder autistic spectrum. While more studies are needed, the results were extremely positive.

KETO DIET AND CANCER

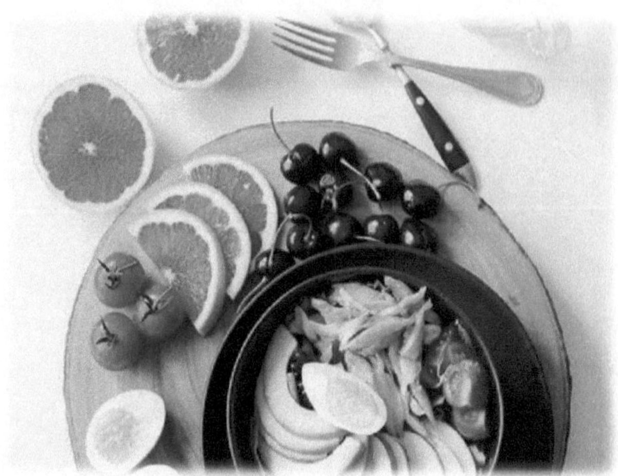

Keto Diet and Cancer

Cancer has turned into a serious disease in our modern society. While cancer was not a large factor before the 20th century (it did exist, of course), our modern diet and sedentary lifestyle have made cancer the second primary cause of death, with 1600 American dying from this disease every day. It appears that our bodies do not react well to being exposed to daily toxins.

While any cancer treatment must be guided by your physician, it is a good idea to discuss the keto diet and what it can do to help in the treatment of this disease.

A cancer-specific keto diet may consist of as much as 90 percent fat. There is a very good reason for that. What doctors do know is that cancer cells feed off carbohydrates and sugar. This is what helps them grow and multiply in number.

As we have seen, the keto diet dramatically reduces our carbohydrate and sugar consumption as our metabolism is altered. What the keto diet does, in essence, is remove the "food" on which

may die, multiply at a slower rate, or decrease.

Another reason why a keto diet is able to slow down the growth of cancer cells is that by reducing calories, cancer cells have less energy to develop and grow in the first place. Insulin also helps cells grow. Since the keto diet lowers insulin level, it slows down the growth of tumorous cells.

When on the keto diet, the body produces ketones. While the body is fueled by ketones, cancerous cells are not. Therefore, a state of ketosis may help reduce the size and growth of cancer cells.

One study monitored the growth of tumors in patients suffering from cancer of the digestive tract. Of those patients who received a high carbohydrate diet, tumors showed a 32.2 percent in growth. Patients on a keto diet showed a 24.3 percent growth in their tumor. The difference is quite significant.
Another study involved five patients who combined chemotherapy with a keto diet. Three of these patient went into remission. Two patients saw a progression of the disease when they went off the keto diet.

More studies are needed, but these numbers are encouraging.

The keto diet may help prevent cancer from occurring in diabetic patients in the first place. People with diabetes have a higher risk level to develop cancer due to elevated blood sugar levels. Since the ketogenic diet is extremely effective at decreasing the levels of blood sugar, it may prevent the initial onset of cancer.

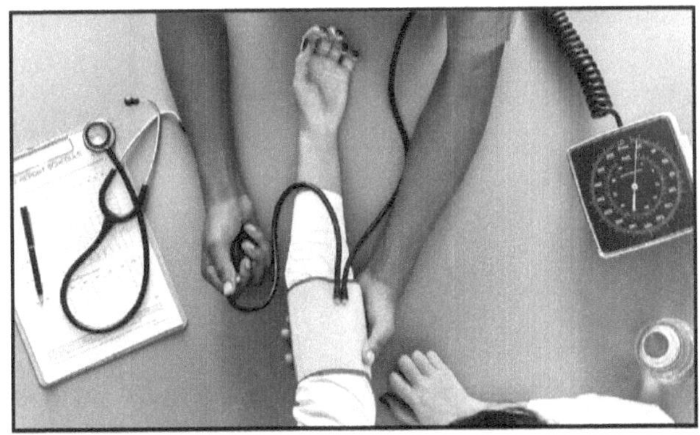

From what research has discovered so far, ketogenic diet may:

1. Stop the growth of cancer cells.

2. Help replace cancerous cells with healthy cells.

3. Change the body's metabolism and enable the body to "starve" cancer cells by depriving them of needed nutrition.

4. By lowering the body's insulin level, the ketogenic body may prevent the onset of cancer cells.

On a ketogenic diet specifically for cancer, your fats should be 75 to 90 percent, protein 15-20 percent, and less than 5 percent carbohydrates.

Foods to Eat

1. Egg, including yolks
2. All green, leafy vegetables, as well as cauliflower, avocado, mushrooms, peppers, cucumbers, and tomatoes.
3. When choosing dairy, opt for full-fat version of cheeses, butter, sour cream, yogurt, and milk.

Eat nuts such as walnuts, almonds, filberts, and sunflower and pumpkin seeds.

Foods to Eat in Moderation

1. Have one serving of root vegetables, such as yams, parsnip, carrots, and turnips per day.
2. Fruits contain sugar, so treat them like candy. One small piece per day.
3. A glass of dry wine, vodka, whiskey and brandy once a week. No cocktails with sugars.
4. A small piece of chocolate with 75 percent or higher cocoa content once a week.

5. Foods to Avoid

1. Any food containing sugar, including cereals; soft drinks, juices, and sports drinks, candies, and chocolate. Limit artificial sweeteners as much as possible.
2. Starchy food such as pasta and potatoes, breads, potato chips, and french fries, cooking oils, and margarine.
3. All beers.

Keto Diet and Epilepsy

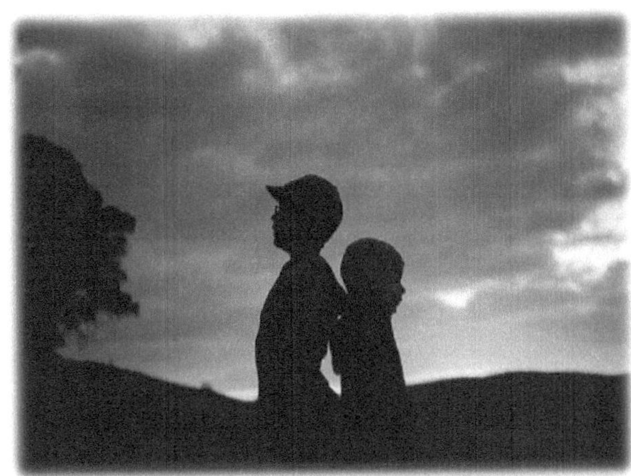

Keto Diet and Epilepsy

The initial use of the keto diet had nothing to do with weight loss or diabetes management, for which it is now so well-known. Instead, the diet was created by a doctor in 1924 to help his patients suffering from epilepsy.

Epilepsy is a nervous system disorder that can bring on recurrent seizures at any time. The symptoms can be spasms and convulsions, or an unusual psychological view of the world. In any case, it is caused by abnormal brain activity. The severity of the symptoms varies from person to person. A person is diagnosed with epilepsy only if he or she suffers from more than two seizures in one full day. Anyone can suffer from this disorder, but it seems to affect young children the most, perhaps because the young brain is still in a state of development.

Seizures are frequently managed by drugs. Sometimes they work; sometimes, they don't.

As far back as 1924, however, Dr. Russell Wilder of the Mayo Clinic conducted groundbreaking research and created the ketogenic diet to help children suffering from epilepsy. It was remarkably effective, but doctors lost interest when new anti-seizure medications came on the market. It was easier for them to prescribe medication than to discuss diet.

However, people who used the keto diet to treat seizures continued seeing remarkable success. Today, doctors are returning to using the low carbohydrate, high-fat diet to treat their patients. The results have been extremely promising.

In 1998, the Journal of Pediatrics published a study involving 150 children who experienced seizures despite taking popular anti-seizure medications. The children were placed on the ketogenic diet for one year which the researchers assessed their progress.

Eighty-three percent of the subjects were still in the study after 3 months. Over one-third of the children showed a 90 percent decrease in seizures. At the end of the year, slightly more than half of the subjects had remained on the diet, and a quarter of them experienced a 90 percent decrease in seizures. The numbers indicate that the keto diet has a tremendously positive effect on children who suffer from seizures. The researchers consider it more effective than medication in many cases.

For anyone with children who experience seizures, the inclusion of a keto diet in the child's treatment should be discussed with his or her physician.

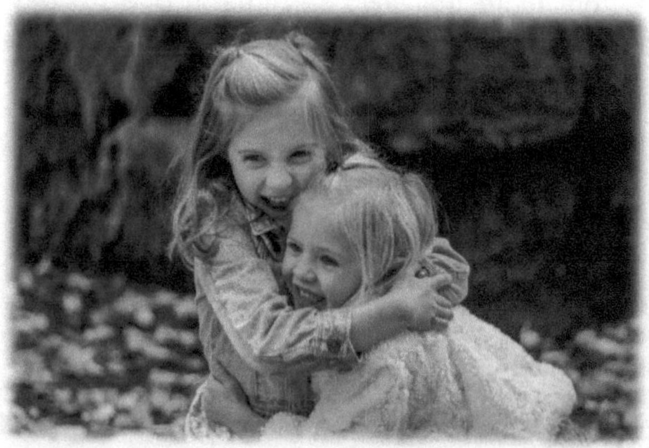

Another research on the effects of the keto diet on childhood epilepsy involved 145 children. The children were divided into two groups, with one group being treated with medication while the other group receiving a ketogenic diet. Seventy-four percent of the ketogenic diet group were successful in reducing seizures.

There have been more studies of childhood epilepsy and the keto diet. These have sparked new and considerable interest within the medical profession.

Keto Diet and Blood Pressure

One-third of American adults suffer from high blood pressure. It is a serious health problem that can lead to heart attacks and strokes. Obviously, the higher the blood pressure, the greater the risk. Aging and obesity greatly increase the chances of developing high blood pressure.

Blood pressure is usually treated with a variety of medications, some of which can have side effects. The best blood pressure is 120/80. High blood pressure is the result of hypertension, and the causes aren't always clear, but we live in an increasingly tense world, and more and more people are dealing with high blood pressure.

It is a known fact that people suffering from high blood pressure frequently carry excess belly fat and can become at risk for type 2 diabetes. To get at the root of all these problems may require a change in lifestyle.

The symptoms of high blood pressure can be caused by an overload of carbohydrates in the diet, more than the body is able to handle. As we've discussed, carbohydrates are converted into sugars, which raise the body's blood sugar level, forcing the body to create additional insulin. Insulin stores fat, and an excess of insulin can lead to obesity. All of this can have a negative effect on your blood pressure.

Consuming fewer carbohydrates decreases both the level of insulin and the blood pressure level. This simple dietary change can make a huge difference in your blood pressure.

In an interesting study released in the Archives of Internal Medicine, 146 overweight people took part in a weight-loss experiment. The people were divided into two groups. One group was put on a ketogenic diet containing a maximum of 20 grams of carbohydrates, while the other group was given the weight-loss drug orlistat, in addition to being counseled to follow a low-fat regimen.
Both groups showed similar weight loss. What surprised the researchers was that half of the keto group showed a decrease in blood pressure, while only 21 percent of the low-fat diet group had any decrease in blood pressure. While weight loss itself would bring about a lowering of blood pressure, the study suggests that a decrease in carbohydrate intake can help lower blood pressure even more.

It was found that potassium specifically had a huge effect on lower hypertension. Doctors recommend at least 4,700 mg of potassium each day for anyone wishing to lower his or her blood pressure.

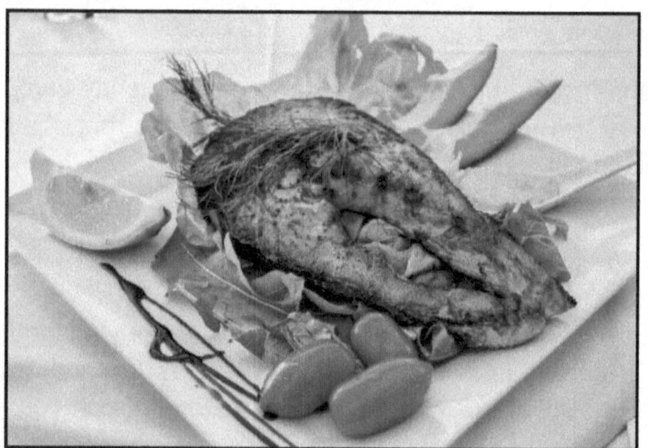

Foods high in potassium are:

- Avocado
- Acorn squash
- Bananas
- Coconut water
- Dried apricots
- Pomegranate
- Salmon
- Spinach
- Sweet potato
- White beans

While all these foods are permitted on the ketogenic diet, limit your intake of sweet potato and beans, which are starchy and can contain a high level of carbs.

What Do I Eat on a Keto Diet?

What Do I Eat on a Keto Diet?

Some people associate the keto diet with the bad word "fat," and are quick to dismiss it. Nothing could be further from the truth. Fat is allowed, because it is converted into energy. Our body needs healthy fats to thrive. Other foods on the diet could not be healthier. When you're eating ketogenic, you're filling your body with nutrition. Let's take a look at the foods you'll be eating.

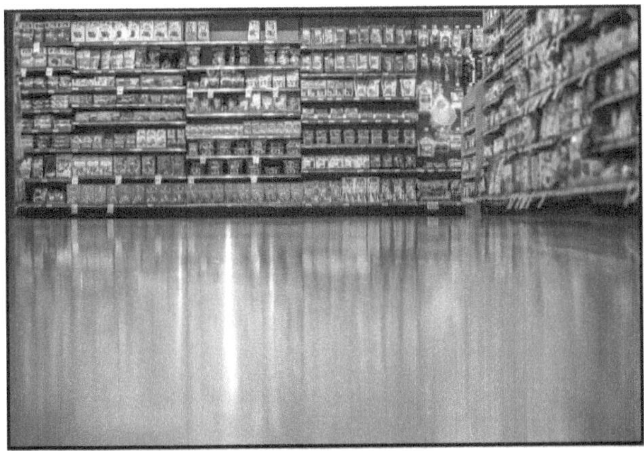

As this book has already pointed out, the elimination of processed foods and sugar is one of the best things you can do for your health in general. Processed foods are filled with toxic preservatives that do nothing for you but rob you of your good health. Fresh is always better. When purchasing anything at the market, get into the habit of reading labels. They can be very sneaky and revealing.

Keep your carbohydrates under 50 grams a day, and you'll feel the difference. A stricter ketogenic diet will contain approximately 20 grams of carbs a day.

Food to Eat on a Ketogenic Diet

1. Seafood

Everyone knows about the healthy fatty acids, vitamins and minerals in seafood. Very few of us eat enough. The keto diet encourages the consumption of all things from the sea. Shrimp and crabs are carb-free, and other shellfish contain only a low amount of carbohydrates.

Fatty fish, such as salmon and sardines, are highly recommended because of their high omega-fatty acid content. Fish truly is brainfood. Enjoy at least two servings or more of seafood a week on the keto diet. Simple canned tuna counts as seafood.

Vegetables

Can a diet that recommends unlimited green, leafy vegetables be anything but healthy? They are extremely low in carbohydrates and bursting with vitamins, antioxidants, and the fiber we need daily. Green vegetables such as broccoli, spinach, and kale are believed to decrease the risk of heart diseases and cancer. Cauliflower and turnips can be prepared to look and taste like rice or mashed potatoes, with much less starch and carbohydrates.

"Starchy" vegetables, such as potatoes or beets do have carbs and should be limited on the keto diet.

3. Dairy Foods

a.　　There are cheeses to satisfy everyone's taste. They are high in fat content for energy, high in protein and calcium, and low in carbohydrates.

b.　　Yogurt and cottage cheese are a great source of protein and calcium. They are low-carb and fit well into the ketogenic lifestyle. Be sure to stick with plain yogurt, as the flavored types contain a lot of sugar, as are the so-called "low fat" versions of yogurt. You can flavor yogurt and cottage cheese yourself with a few berries and nuts.

4. Avocados

Avocados are truly "superfood." They are high in important vitamins and minerals, including potassium. According to a study, avocados are also believed to help lower cholesterol by 22 percent.

Loaded with nutrients and delicious taste, avocados only have 2 grams of net carbohydrates. Use them in salads and sandwiches.

5. Meat and Poultry

The keto diet lets you eat plenty of meat. Meat contains very few carbs and is high in protein to help you build muscles. Whenever possible, choose healthy, grass-fed meats, which are higher in fatty acids.

6. Eggs

Eggs are high in protein and contain a mere 1 gram of carbohydrates. As they are also inexpensive, they are ideal for anyone on a ketogenic diet.

Eggs also make you feel full, thereby helping you eat less. Many people take pride in only consuming the whites of eggs, but the true nutrition lies in the yolk, so be sure to eat the egg in its entirety.

7. Coconut Oil

Too many people are unfamiliar with coconut oil, another "superfood." It is perfect for people dealing with diabetes and has been used with Alzheimer patients.

Coconut oil can be used in most recipes in place of butter or oil. You can also use it for frying and sautéing.

8. Dark Chocolate

Did you know that dark chocolate has a high amount of antioxidants? As a matter of fact, dark chocolate is reaching superfood status. Chocolate with 80 percent or higher real cocoa powder can lower your blood pressure.

An ounce of 80 percent dark chocolate contains 10 grams of carbohydrates, so it definitely counts as a healthy snack. Keep in mind the lower of cocoa content, the less healthy the chocolate will be. Milk chocolate does not count as a healthy chocolate.

The keto diet has a lot less restricted foods than many other diets. Sugar, of course, should be avoided. That doesn't mean you can't enjoy sweet desserts. There are many keto-friendly recipes that substitute unsweetened apple sauce for sugar in baked goods. Substitute sweeteners such as Stevia can also be used in moderation.

Keep in mind that fruits are healthful, but they do contain a great deal of sugar, so limit the amount you eat to just a few slices a day. Fruit juices are concentrates that have vitamins but lack fiber. And their sugar content is extremely high. Read the label on any bottle of juice before buying. The best juices are "green" with just a hint of fruit for flavoring.

Be careful with cereals. Most are packed with sugar and robbed of any nutrients. Many claim, "nutrition added," but all that means is that all nutrition has been removed and replaced with a small amount, and a whole lot of sugar for taste. One hundred percent bran cereal will fit into your keto diet, and you can sweeten it with a handful of berries. Just be sure to examine all labels in the cereal aisle. They can be very tricky. Also, remember that honey, too, is considered as sugar.

Totally omit white starches from your diet. They are nothing but empty calories. This includes white bread, pasta, and rice. Buy the wholegrain version, instead, and enjoy in moderation.

Legumes and beans are healthy for you, but they are high in carbohydrates. You can have them occasionally; just make sure you keep it within your daily 20 – 5o carb-gram count.

Alcohols tend to be empty calories, but certain spirits will be better for you than others. Beer is filled with carbs and should be off your keto diet. The expression "beer belly" exists for a reason. Enjoy a glass of wine, instead. Of course, there are variances in different types wine. Dry wines contain a minimum amount of sugar, while sweet dessert wines contain much more.

Pure alcohol such as whiskey and vodka are carb-free, but they do contain calories, so have a care. Mixing alcohol for fancy cocktails usually creates a haven for sugar, so avoid those.

Wine coolers may be a tasty treat, but in reality, they are just sugary sodas with some added alcohol. They should definitely not be on your keto diet at any time.

Keto Diet For Rapid Weight Loss

Many people confuse the ketogenic diet with low carb diets or paleo diets. However, there are considerable differences of which you should be aware.

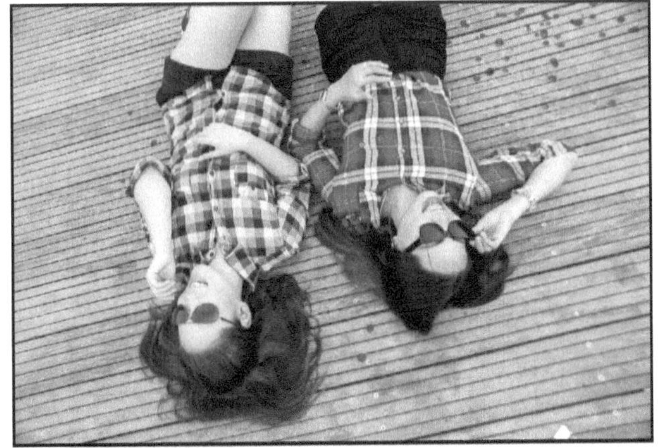

Keto v. Low Carb

A low-carb diet can be anything it wants to be, as long as it is low in carbohydrates. And "low" is rarely defined. On a low-carb diet, you simply make random food choices that curb your carb intake arbitrarily. Since there is no real number, you might still be consuming too many carbs.

Most importantly, what the low-carb diet lacks is that all-critical ketonic state that turns carbs into fats and provides your body with a new and effective source of fuel. This can leave you very hungry and tired.

The ketogenic diet has a specific ratio of carbs to fats to protein. This manipulation is critical, and it's why a low carb diet won't work as well, if at all.

Keto v. Paleo

The Paleo is also a low-carb-type diet. It is based on the assumption that eating the way our cavemen ancestors did, i.e., meat and no carbs, sugars, or grains, is the healthiest type of diet.

There are problems with this reasoning. First, our ancestors never experienced the kind of diseases that we face. The ketogenic diet is specifically a "healing" diet that is meant to benefit the body in many ways and help prevent diseases. The paleo diet does not do that.

Also, the paleo diet is based on eating meat instead of manipulating the ratio of fats, carbohydrates, and protein to achieve a ketonic state that uses fat as fuel.

Ketogenic Diet

Basically, ketogenic is low-carb, but it is much more.

There is a reason the ketogenic diet has become so popular. It helps improve your overall wellbeing in addition to helping you lose weight. You have more energy during the day, and you feel sated and full, thereby reducing the cravings for unhealthy snacks. In essence, you are eating less, but better. That's what makes the keto diet so unique and successful.

The ketogenic diet is not magic pill made up by some gurus. Countless studies and testimonials are able to back the effectiveness of this diet. It is a scientifically proven method that balances your body's fat intake to help achieve optimal weight loss.

By using fat instead of sugar as your primary source of energy, the keto diet induces a state of ketosis, which is achieved when your body stops receiving carbohydrates to turn in glucose. The fewer carbohydrates you consume, the more you force your body to burn fat for energy instead of storing it.

This is why it is possible to lose weight so quickly on the keto diet. It counts carbohydrates instead of calories. Using fats as an additional energy source is what ketosis is all about. It is a natural state that helped our hunter-gatherer ancestors survive in early days.

They feasted on low-carb foods when they could, and fasted when food was scarce. Fat was stored and converted into energy during the scarce times. The ketogenic state is a natural human state, which makes the ketogenic diet so powerful and successful. In addition to the benefits of the keto diet, most people simply enjoy the way it makes them feel better.

Weight loss results on the keto diet differ among individuals, depending on their specific body composition. But weight loss has been the consistent result of people who've been on the keto diet. The keto diet is known as the best weight-loss diet, as well as the healthiest.

A 2017 study divided Crossfit-training subjects into two groups, with both groups following the physical training, but only one group combined the ketogenic diet with the training. The results showed that those on the keto diet decreased their fat mass and weight far more than the other group.

The keto diet group showed an average of 3.5 kilo weight loss, 2.6 percent of body fat, and 2.83 kilos in fat mass, while the other group lost no weight, body fat or fat mass. Both groups showed similar athletic performance ability.

A 2012 study divided overweight children and adolescents into two group; one was put on a keto diet, the other on a low-calorie diet. As in other keto studies, the children on the keto diet decreased their weight, fat mass, and lowered their insulin levels considerably more than the low-calorie group.

Besides more rapid weight loss, a decided advantage of the keto diet over a low-calorie diet is that people actually stick to the keto diet. A low-calorie diet will help you lose weight, but you may be constantly feeling hungry and deprived. That is the main reason most diets fail. Hunger and deprivation are not a part of the ketogenic lifestyle.

Ketosis Explained

As we have stated earlier, the keto diet isn't magic. It is proven science. Ketosis is a natural occurrence that happens when you don't feed your body enough carbohydrates and it is forced to look for energy elsewhere.

You have undoubtedly experienced ketosis when you've missed a meal or have exhausted your body with rigorous exercise. Whenever these things happen, your body helps you out by raising its level of ketones. However, most people eat enough sugar and carbs to keep ketosis from happening.
We love our sugar and carbs, no matter how bad they are for us, and our bodies will happily use them as fuel. And since our bodies want to help us out, it turns any excess glucose into fat and stores it for future use. Stored fat translated into those ridiculous belly fat that you never want.

The more you restrict your carbohydrate consumption, the more your body will produce ketones. It really has no other options. When we restrict the amount of carbohydrates that we eat, our body will still provide us with energy, but it must turn to another source. And that alternate source is fat that was so thoughtfully stored for emergencies. The result is a state of ketosis. It happens when our body breaks down the fat into fatty acids and glycerol.

Researchers have discovered most of what they know about ketosis from people who fast, thereby depriving them of all sources of energy. After two days of fasting, the body is starting to produce ketones as it breaks down the available protein and begins to use stored fat for fuel. Ketosis is the natural process the body goes through when deprived of other sources of energy.

Obviously, going on a ketogenic diet is healthier than fasting. Ketogenic should become a lifestyle, not a quick weight-loss method. One of the reasons it is so beneficial is that ketones offer protection against diseases and damages that can affect the body.

Getting Started on the Keto Diet

You're ready for a new and improved you. Congratulations. There are so many wonderful benefits to the ketogenic diet, you can expect many positive changes, both physical and mental. So, let's not delay and get the journey started.

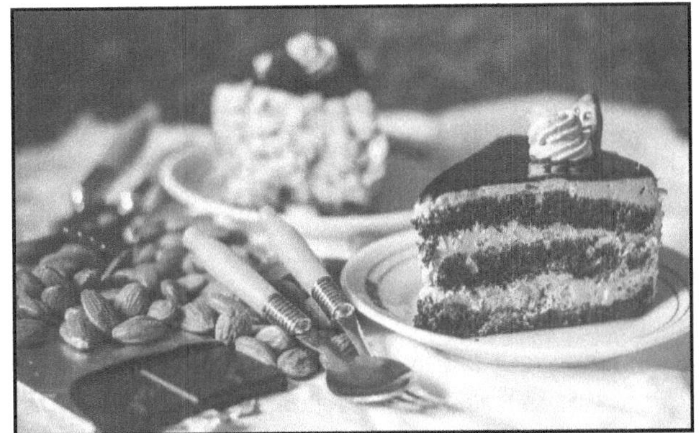

Clear Your Pantry

We're sure you have plenty of willpower, but there is no need to confront a kitchen filled with tempting sugars and carbohydrates. Make a clean sweep and pack the offending items in a box. Then donate the loot to a needy neighbor or a soup kitchen. They will appreciate your gesture, and you are on your way to a keto lifestyle. If you have family, try to get them involved. If they refuse to refrain from eating carbs and sugar, at least insist they do so away from home. It's a fair request.

Weigh Yourself

The keto diet does not require you to live by the tyranny of the scale. As a matter of fact, as you build up healthy muscles, you might notice a slight initial gain. That's great, so don't worry.

You should, however, have an idea of what your starting point is. If you opted for the keto diet solely to lose weight, you'll be able to track your progress. But don't become a slave to the scale. The occasional weigh-in, perhaps once a week, is enough.

What About Your Favorite Meals?

Perhaps the very thought of giving up your favorite foods has prevented you from getting started on the keto way of life. Relax. The truth is, for every dish that you love and can't live without (yes, that includes cheesecake and mashed potatoes!), you can easily find a low-carb substitute that is just as tasty.

First, let's consider items at your market labeled "low carbohydrate." Labels are frustratingly deceiving, and you'd have to be a nutritional expert to understand them. All-too-frequently, off-the-shelf low carb products have simply substituted sugar for carbs, so don't fall for that bit of deceit. You need to learn to read labels with the diligence that you'd read your wealthy uncle's will, but your best bet is to stay away from these products and simply find healthier substitutes. The same goes for anything labeled "low fat," which inevitably means added sugars.

Craving a taco? Use a lettuce wrap instead of a taco shell. Do you want rice or mashed potatoes? Grate or rice a cauliflower, and you won't be able to tell the difference. Can't give up your favorite pasta dish? Turn a zucchini into "zoodles" by slicing it or using a spiral cutter and enjoy your pasta. You absolutely have to have your favorite dessert? On the keto diet, you can. Just bake with almond flour and use unsweetened applesauce and/or avocado to create some sweet smoothness.

Learn about coconut oil, which can be used as a butter substitute in sautéing, frying, and baking. Coconut oil has incredible health benefits, especially for Type-2 diabetics.

On the keto diet, you'll be able to enjoy all your favorite meals, only better.

Always Stay Hydrated

The keto diet tends to lower your insulin level, so your kidneys may be excreting more liquid than usual. Be sure to drink plenty of water.

Condiments Can Be the Enemy

Don't assume condiments don't count on a diet. On the keto diet, they most certainly do. Ketchup is filled with sugar. Not all salad dressings are equal. Read the label, and never opt for the "fat-free" version. They have merely substituted sugar for fat. Ordering salads when eating out is one of your best options, but beware of the dressing that the restaurant serves. Either ask about the ingredients, or better, bring your own salad dressing. Don't hesitate to do that, even in a posh eatery where the Maître d' might become spastic at the sight of you pulling salad dressing out of your bag.

Keep Track of Your Ketone Level

It's especially important to remain aware of how your body is responding to the keto diet at the start of the diet. You can do so by doing a simple urine test. You can also purchase a blood ketone meter. It is recommened to perform the test early in the morning.

Friends and Family Can Be Annoying – Bless Their Hearts

Those nearest and dearest to you may not always understand what you are doing. When eating as a group, they may put subtle pressure on you to "just try a bite," or "one slice of cake won't kill you." Or worse, "but I cooked it especially for you!"

It will take resolve to stick to your diet. It may help to fill up on keto-friendly snacks before you sit down and eat. Enjoy some nuts, an avocado, or just a leg of chicken *before* you eat, and you will be less tempted.

Celebrate!

Celebratory occasions, especially if you're the guest of honor, can be a huge hurdle. When the gang at the office or your parents enter a room with a cake yelling "Surprise!" on your birthday, it's hard to refuse. So, try being a bit sneaky, instead.

By all means gush over the offering. You are expected to do that. You can even help cut slices. Then, discover a sudden and irresistible urge for coffee, which you verbalize loudly and clearly. Gently remove yourself from the center of activity to get coffee for yourself and anyone else. By the time anyone notices, hopefully they've missed the fact that you haven't eaten anything.

Traveling

Traveling while on the keto diet can be a challenge, so be prepared. Pack a personal blender with some avocados and bananas for a few quick and healthful smoothies. Pack some anchovies or tuna for protein.

Eating Out

Eating out isn't as difficult as you may think. Even fast-food places have salads, these days. In any restaurant, stick to meat and vegetables and forego the potatoes and noodles.

You can even navigate the tricky maze in a Chinese restaurant. While abstaining from rice, you can enjoy the following: clear soups, steamed fish with vegetables, egg foo young, stir-fried dishes, Mu Shu without the wrappers are just a few suggestions. Ask your server if your meal can be prepared without cornstarch which is frequently used as a thickener.

Even if you end up in a fast food place that doesn't have salad, simply toss the buns from your burger and just eat the meat. You can do the same at a friend's house or at a BBQ.

Exercise

The keto diet will build muscle mass and give you added energy. Don't forget to incorporate exercise into your daily routine. It can be as simple as walking more, taking the stairs, or joining a gym.

How Long Should You Stay on a Ketogenic Diet"

The amount of time spent on the diet can vary and should be discussed with your doctor. Many people who use the ketogenic diet for weight loss remain on the diet for several weeks, until they have achieved a goal, then they turn to a paleo diet or other maintenance eating. You do not want to lose weight only to return to your old eating habits.

If you are on the ketogenic diet for medical or therapeutic reasons, check with your doctor to ascertain if you should remain on the diet for a longer period of time.

Keto Recipes

You can take your favorite recipes and turned them "keto." Below are a few recipes to show you how easy it is. It might be an excellent idea to buy a keto cookbook for your kitchen.

Two of the most important keto recipes are the simple cauliflower rice and "zoodles." They couldn't be easier to prepare. People can get frustrated on the keto diet when they crave pasta and rice. These two recipes definitely satisfy those cravings; they taste just like the real thing. The zoodles can be used for any pasta dish.

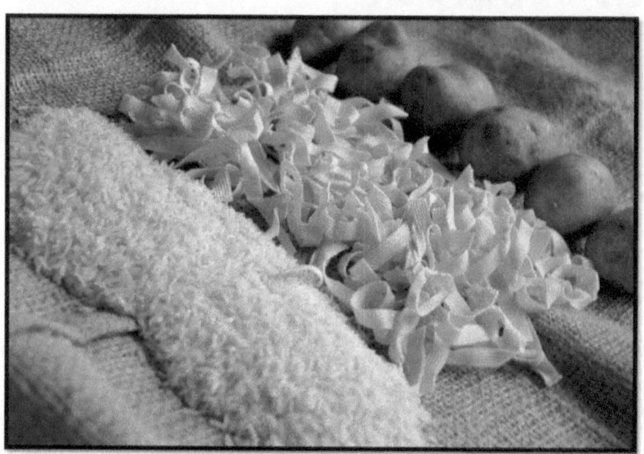

KETO RECIPES

45. KETO CHEESEBURGER
46. DESSERT RECIPES
47. CAKE
48. CHEESECAKE KETO FAT BOMBS
49. KETO BROWNIES
50. KETO ICE CREAM
51. KETO EGG CREPES
52. KETO NAAN
53. PEANUT BUTTER COOKIES
54. BUTTERY KETO CREPES
55. KETO LEMON FAT BOMB
56. PEANUT BUTTER BALLS
57. NUT FREE KETO BROWNIE
58. SMOOTIES
59. COFFEE SMOOTHIE
60. CHAI PUMPKIN SMOOTHIE
61. CASHEW SMOOTHIE
62. BREAKFAST SMOOTHIE
63. KETO MILKSHAKE SMOOTHIE
64. AVOCADO SMOOTHIE
65. COLLAGEN SMOOTHIE
66. FAT BOMB SMOOTHIE
67. CINNAMON SMOOTHIE
68. KETO ICE CREAM
69. KETO EGG CREPES
70. KETO NAAN
71. PEANUT BUTTER COOKIES
72. BUTTERY KETO CREPES
73. KETO LEMON FAT BOMB
74. PEANUT BUTTER BALLS
75. NUT FREE KETO BROWNIE
76. SMOOTIES
77. COFFEE SMOOTHIE
78. CHAI PUMPKIN SMOOTHIE
79. CASHEW SMOOTHIE
80. BREAKFAST SMOOTHIE
81. KETO MILKSHAKE SMOOTHIE
82. AVOCADO SMOOTHIE
83. COLLAGEN SMOOTHIE
84. FAT BOMB SMOOTHIE
85. CINNAMON SMOOTHIE
86. TROPICAL SMOOTHIE

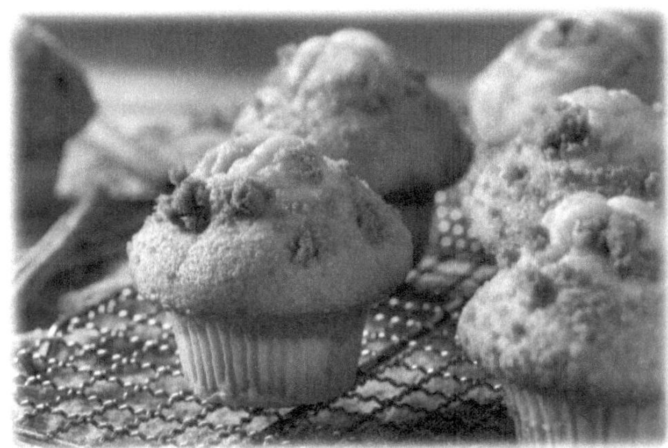

KETO BREAKFAST MUFFINS

Serves: 6-8
Prep Time: 10 Minutes
Cook Time: 15 Minutes
Total Time: 25 Minutes
INGREDIENTS
-        3 tablespoons plain Keto& Hot breakfast cereal
-        3 eggs
-        2 tablespoons heavy cream
-        2 tablespoons flaxseed meal
-        3 tablespoons coconut oil
-        2 tablespoons Erythritol
-        1 tsp vanilla extract
-        1 tsp baking powder

DIRECTIONS
Preheat oven to 325 F
In a bowl mix Plain keto & Hot breakfast cereal, add
coconut oil and mix well.
Add the rest of ingredients and mix
Pour batter into 6-8 cupcakes and bake for 15-18 minutes
Remove and serve.

KETO PANCAKES

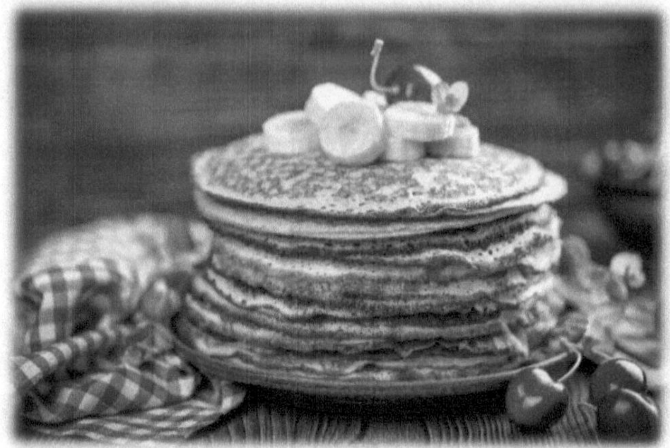

Serves: 4
Prep Time: 10 Minutes
Cook Time: 10 Minutes
Total Time: 20 Minutes
INGREDIENTS
-        1/2 cup almond flour
-        3 eggs
-        1/2 tsp cinnamon
-        1 tablespoon butter
-        1/2 cup cream cheese

DIRECTIONS
Place all ingredients in a bowl and mix using a
blender
In a frying pan pour 2-3 tablespoons of pancake
mixture and cook for 1-2 minutes per side
Remove and top with cinnamon or butter.

BREAKFAST SANDWICH

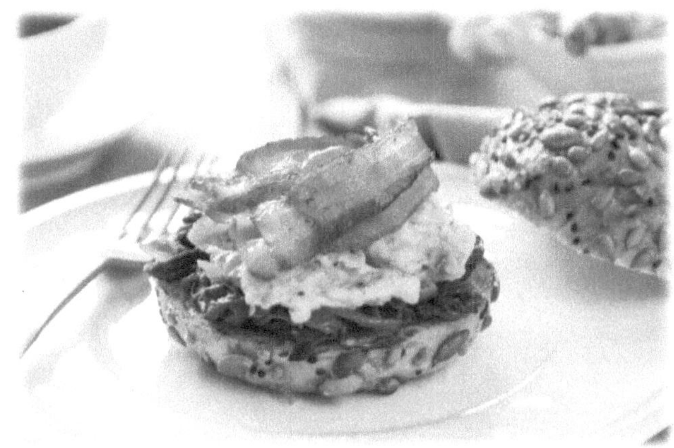

Serves: 1
Prep Time: 5 Minutes
Cook Time: 5 Minutes
Total Time: 10 Minutes
INGREDIENTS
-        3 tablespoons shredded cheddar cheese
-        1 egg
-        1 slice bacon
-        salt

DIRECTIONS
In a skillet add shredded cheese oven medium heat
and remove to a paper towel when it starts to melt
Cook the egg as you want, place it over the cheese and
season with salt
Place the remaining cheese over the top and serve.

POWER BREAKFAST WITH GREEN SAUCE

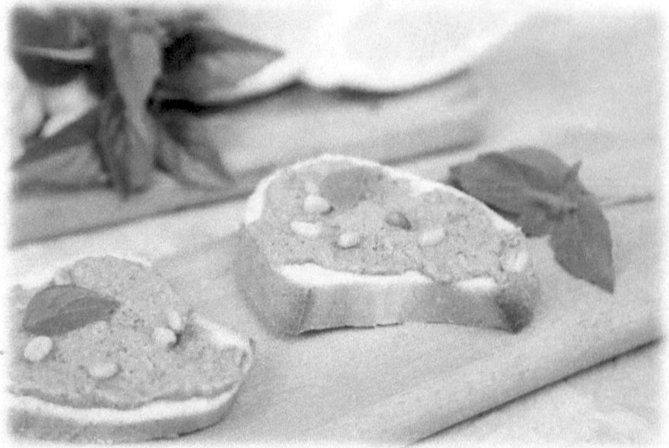

Serves: 3
Prep Time: 10 Minutes
Cook Time: 10 Minutes
Total Time: 20 Minutes
INGREDIENTS
-        1 cup baby spinach
- salt
-        1 cup parsley
-        4 garlic cloves
-        4 tablespoons hemp hearts
-        1 cup olive oil
-        4 slices bacon
-        1 cup arugula
-        1 egg
-        10 asparagus tips
DIRECTIONS
1. For Green Sauce mix arugula, olive oil, parsley, garlic cloves, baby spinach, hemp hearts in a blender and blend until smooth
Arrange bacon sliced into rings and place the bacon in the oven at 325 F and cook until done
Tuck 3-4 asparagus tips into each bacon ring and add green sauce, sprinkle salt and pepper and cook for another 12-15 minutes
Remove from oven and serve
PEPPER RINGS

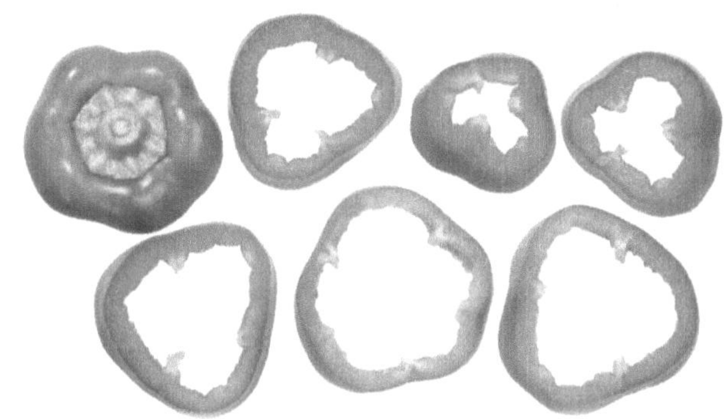

Serves: 2
Prep Time: 10 Minutes
Cook Time: 10 Minutes
Total Time: 20 Minutes

INGREDIENTS

- 2 red bell peppers

- salt

- pepper

- 6 eggs

- 1 lb. breakfast sausage

- 3 tablespoons parmesan cheese

- coconut oil

DIRECTIONS

In a skillet brown breakfast sausage and set aside
Cut peppers into 4-6 rings and place them in the
skillet and cook
Pour the egg into the ring and add salt and sausage
around the yolk of each ring
When ready remove and serve

KETO EGG BITES

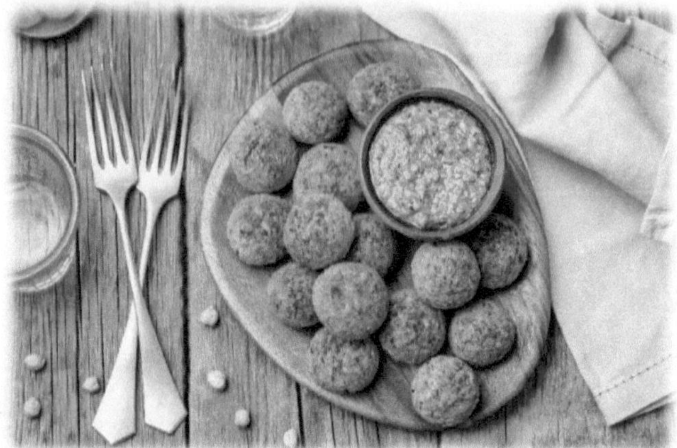

Serves: 2
Prep Time: 10 Minutes
Cook Time: 20 Minutes
Total Time: 30 Minutes
INGREDIENTS
-        4 eggs
-        1/2 cup swiss cheese
-        1/2 cup fat cottage cheese
-        1/2 tsp salt
-        black pepper
-        2 thick slices of paleo sugar free bacon
DIRECTIONS
Preheat oven to 325 F and place a baking dish
In a bowl mix cottage cheese, salt, pepper cheese, eggs
and blend until smooth
Spray a muffin tin and pour the mixture into it, add
chopped bacon and bake for 25 minutes
Remove and serve

BREAKFAST BOWL

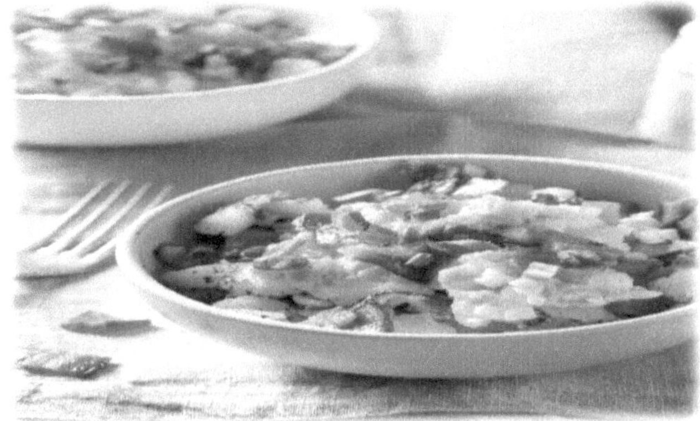

Serves: 1
Prep Time: 10 Minutes
Cook Time: 10 Minutes
Total Time: 20 Minutes
INGREDIENTS
-       2 eggs
-       2 strips bacon
-       1/2 up cheddar cheese
-       1/2 cup salsa
-       2 tablespoons butter
-       1/2 avocado
DIRECTIONS
In a bowl scramble the eggs and place them into the skillet, cook for 2-3 minutes
Top the eggs with shredded cheese and bacon
Slice avocado and place it over the bacon
Top with salsa and serve

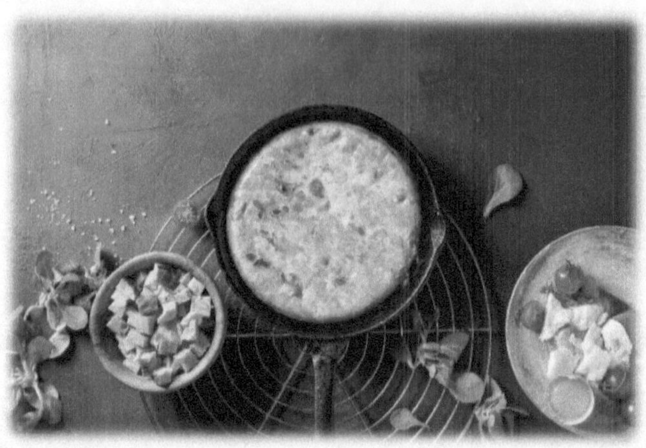

KETO POTATOES

Serves: 4
Prep Time: 10 Minutes
Cook Time: 10 Minutes
Total Time: 20 Minutes
INGREDIENTS

-        1 large turnip

-        1/2 paprika, garlic powder, salt

- parsley

-        1/2 onion

-        2 slices bacon

-        1 tablespoon olive oil

DIRECTIONS

In a skillet add the turnips and spices, cook for 5-6
minutes, add onion and cook for another 2-3 minutes
Chop the bacon and add to the skillet, cook for
another 2-3 minutes
Remove to a place and top with parsley before serving

MINI BREAKFAST MEATLOAFS

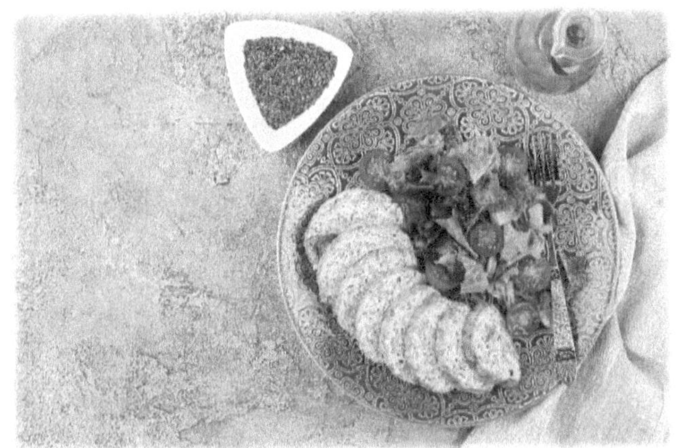

Serves: 4
Prep Time: 10 Minutes
Cook Time: 30 Minutes
Total Time: 40 Minutes
INGREDIENTS
-        1 lb. pork sausage
-        1 egg
-        1 cup shredded cheddar cheese
-        4 slices bacon
-        4 slices ham

DIRECTIONS

Preheat oven to 325 F
In a bowl mix all ingredients
Divide mixture into 6-8 portions and pack into mini
loaf pan cavities
Bake for 30 minutes, remove and serve

KETO JALAPENO MUFFINS

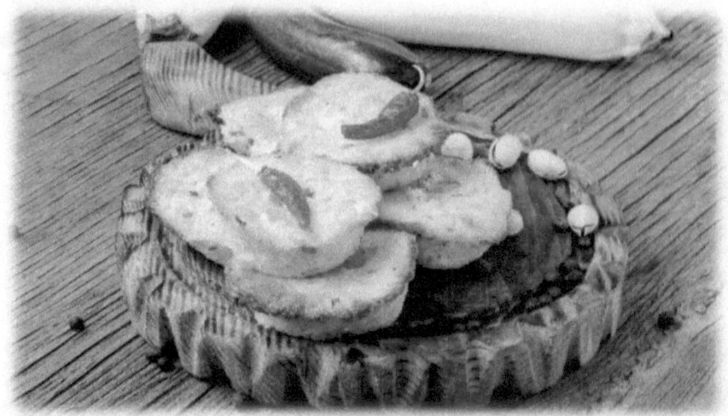

Serves: 4
Prep Time: 10 Minutes
Cook Time: 30 Minutes
Total Time: 40 Minutes

INGREDIENTS
-        8 eggs
-        8 oz. cheese
-        3/4 cup heavy cream
-        salt
-        jalapeno
-        8 slices bacon

DIRECTIONS

Preheat oven to 325
Add bacon to each muffin tin
In a bowl mix cream, cheese, epper, eggs and salt
Distribute into 8-10 muffin cups and add jalapeno to
each muffin tin
Bake for 15-20 minutes, when ready remove and serve
LUNCH RECIPES SOUP RECIPES
KETO BROCCOLI SOUP

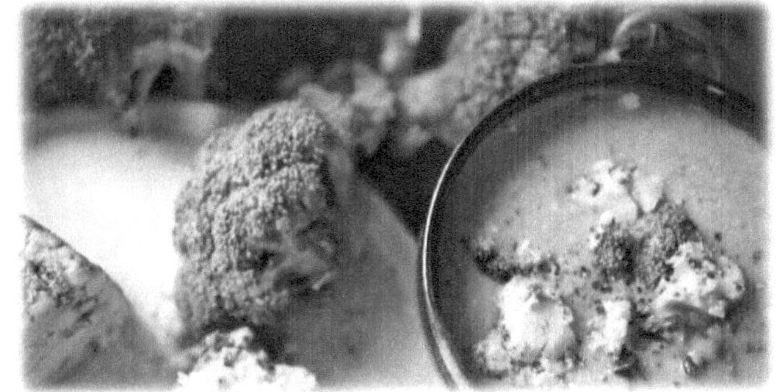

Serves: 4
Prep Time: 10 Minutes
Cook Time: 30 Minutes
Total Time: 40 Minutes

INGREDIENTS
-       olive oil
-       1 cup chicken broth
-       1 cup heavy whipping cream
-       6 oz. shredded cheddar cheese - salt
-       5-ounces broccoli
-       1 celery stalk
-       1 small carrot
-       1/2 onion

DIRECTIONS

In a pot add olive oil over medium heat
Add onion, carrot, celery and cook for 2-3 minutes
Add chicken broth and simmer for 4-5 minutes
Stir in broccoli and cream
Sprinkle in cheese and season with salt

KETO TACO SOUP

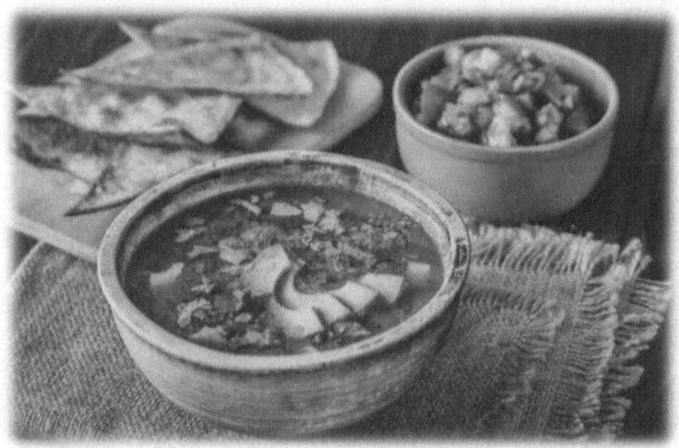

Serves: 8
Prep Time: 10 Minutes
Cook Time: 10 Minutes
Total Time: 20 Minutes

INGREDIENTS

-       2 lbs. ground beef
-       1 onion
-       1 cup heavy whipping cream
-       1 tsp chili powder
-       14 oz. cream cheese
-       1 tsp garlic
-       1 tsp cumin
-       2 10 oz. cans tomatoes
-       16 oz. beef broth

DIRECTIONS

Cook for a couple of minutes, onion, garlic and beef
Add cream cheese and stir until fully melted
Add tomatoes, whipping cream, beef broth, stir and bring to boil

<u>KETO CHICKEN SOUP</u>

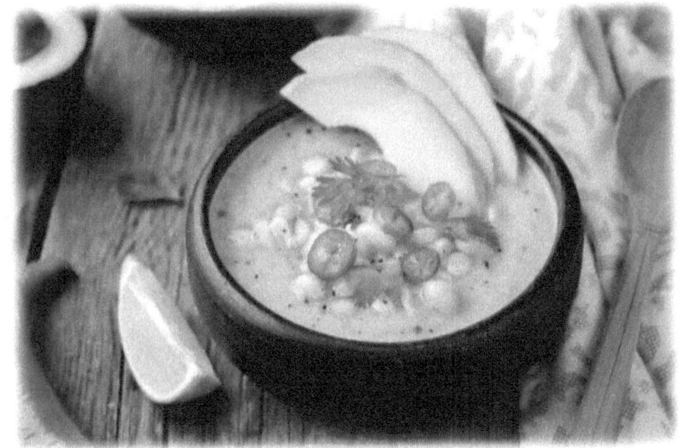

Serves: 4
Prep Time: 10 Minutes
Cook Time: 30 Minutes
Total Time: 40 Minutes

INGREDIENTS

-        2 boneless chicken breast
-        20-ounces diced tomatoes
-        1/2 tsp salt
-        1 cup salsa
-        6-ounces cream cheese
-        avocado
-        2 tablespoons taco seasoning
-        1 cup chicken broth

DIRECTIONS

In a slow cooker place all ingredients and cook for 5-6
hours or until chicken is tender
Whisk cream cheese into the broth
When ready, remove and serve

KETO SPINACH SOUP

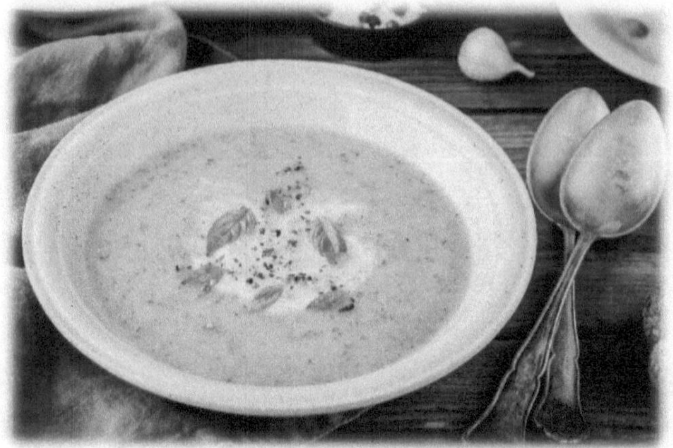

Serves: 2
Prep Time: 5 Minutes
Cook Time: 15 Minutes
Total Time: 20 Minutes

INGREDIENTS

-        1/4 lbs. spinach
-        2 oz. onion
-        1/4 lbs. heavy cream
-        1/2 oz. garlic
-        1 chicken stock cube
-        1,5 cup water
-        1 tablespoons butter

DIRECTIONS

In a saucepan melt the butter and sauté the onion
Add garlic, spinach and stock cube and half the water
Cook until spinach wilts
Pour everything in a blender and blend, add water
Serve with pepper and toasted nuts

KETO TOSCANA SOUP

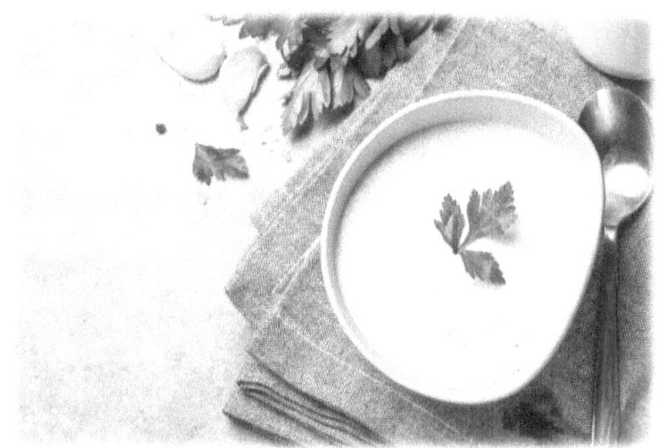

Serves: 4
Prep Time: 10 Minutes
Cook Time: 30 Minutes
Total Time: 40 Minutes

INGREDIENTS

-        1 lb. Italian sausage
-        1/2 cup whipping cream
-        1 tsp garlic
-        2 cup kale leaves
-        1 bag radishes 16-ounces
-        1 onion
-        30-ounces vegetable broth

DIRECTIONS

Cut radishes into small chunks and blend until smooth
In a pot add onion and sausage, cook until brown, add radishes, broth
Cook on medium heat, add heavy whipping cream, kale leaves Cook for a couple minutes
Remove and serve

KETO PARMESAN SOUP

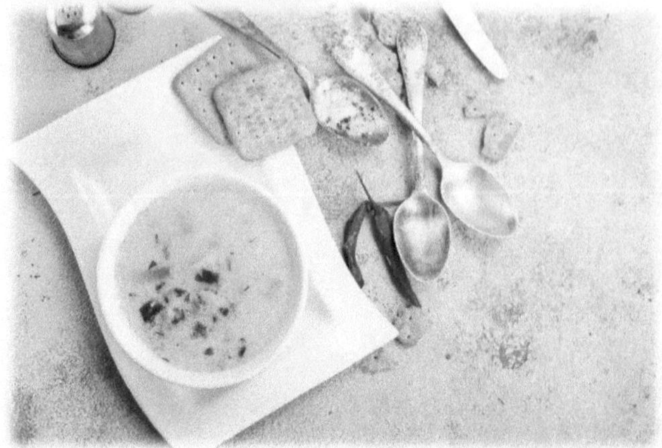

Serves: 4
Prep Time: 10 Minutes
Cook Time: 30 Minutes
Total Time: 40 Minutes

INGREDIENTS
-        1 broccoli
-        1 tsp pepper
-        1 tablespoon butter
-        1 tablespoon cheese
-        1 onion
-        1/2 cup warm
-        1 tsp salt
-        1/2 cup heavy cream

DIRECTIONS

In a saucepan add onion and cook
Stir in broccoli and cook until soft
Combine with heavy cream and place in a blender,
blend until smooth
Return the soup to the saucepan, season with salt
Serve and sprinkle with parmesan.

KETO CAULIFLOWER SOUP

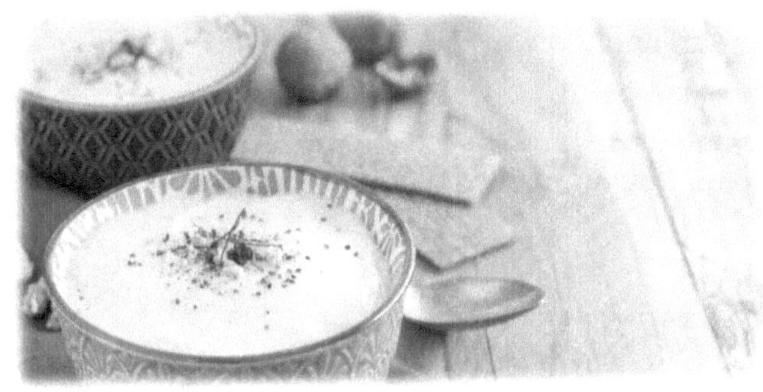

Serves: **4**

Prep Time: **10** Minutes

Cook Time: **30** Minutes

Total Time: **40** Minutes

INGREDIENTS

- $^1/_2$ head of cauliflower
- $^1/_2$ **cup heavy cream**
- $^1/_2$ **red bell pepper**
- **1 tsp salt**
- **1 tsp pepper**
- **1 tablespoon butter**
- **1 tablespoons parmesan cheese**
- **1 tsp herbs**

DIRECTIONS

1. In a saucepan melt butter, add cauliflower and cook until soft
2. Remove from saucepan and set aside
3. Melt butter and sauté and bell pepper
4. In a food processor add cauliflower mixture, pepper and cook for 4-5 minutes
5. Season with salt and pepper
6. Garnish with parmesan and serve

KETO BROCCOLI CHEESE SOUP

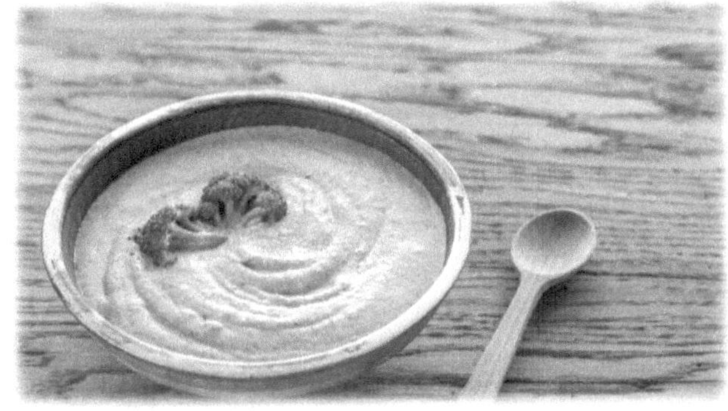

Serves: **2**

Prep Time: **10** Minutes

Cook Time: **20** Minutes

Total Time: **30** Minutes

INGREDIENTS

- 2 cups broccoli
- 3 cups chicken broth
- 1 onion
- 1 cup heavy cream
- 6 oz. cream cheese
- 1 tablespoon hot sauce
- 3 tablespoons butter
- 1 clove garlic
- 6 oz. cheddar cheese

DIRECTIONS

1. In a saucepan melt butter, add onion, garlic and sauté until soft
2. Pour in heavy cream, chicken broth, stir in broccoli
3. Cover and continue cooking for 12-15 minutes
4. Add cheese and cook until melted
5. Stir in hot sauce and enjoy

KETO QUESO SOUP

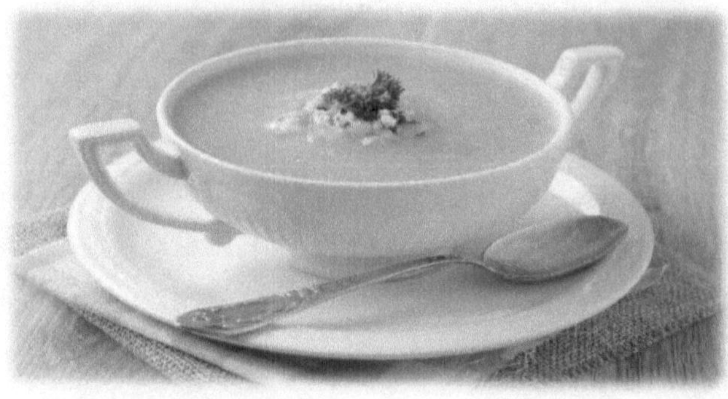

Serves: **4**

Prep Time: **10** Minutes

Cook Time: **30** Minutes

Total Time: **40** Minutes

INGREDIENTS

- 1 lb. chicken breast
- 1 tablespoon taco seasoning
- 1 tablespoon avocado oil
- 1 can diced green chilies
- 6-ounces cream cheese
- $^1/_2$ cup heavy cream
- salt
- 2 cups chicken broth

DIRECTIONS

1. In an iron Dutch oven heat oil over medium heat stir in taco seasoning and cook for 1-2 minutes
2. Add broth, chicken and simmer for 20 minutes, remove chicken and shred
3. Stir in cream cheese and heavy cream into the soup, once the cheese has melted, add the chicken back to the soup, season with salt and serve

KETO SALAD

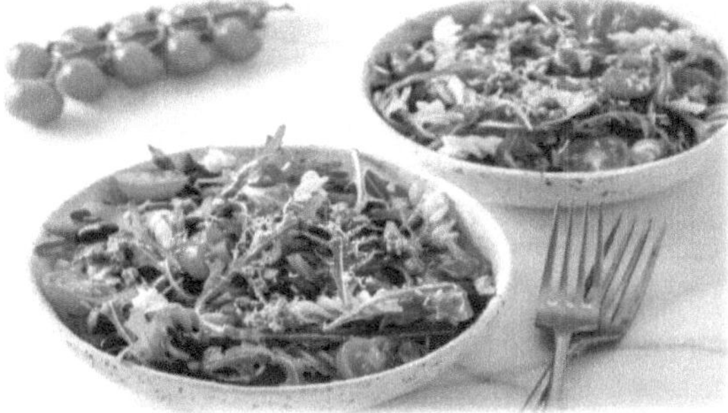

Serves: **2**
Prep Time: **10** Minutes

Cook Time: **10** Minutes

Total Time: **20** Minutes

INGREDIENTS

- 1 slice bacon
- 3-ounces chicken breast
- 1-ounce cheddar cheese
- 1 tablespoon olive oil
- 1 tablespoon apple cider vinegar
- $^1/_2$ avocado
- 1 head romaine lettuce

DIRECTIONS

1. Chop all ingredients and place them in a bowl
2. Mix well and add pepper, oil and vinegar

KETO BROCCOLI SALAD

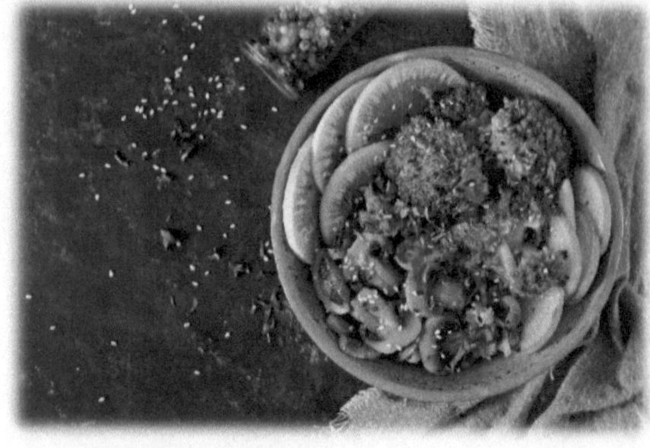

Serves: **2**
Prep Time: **10** Minutes

Cook Time: **10** Minutes

Total Time: **20** Minutes

INGREDIENTS

- 20-ounce raw broccoli
- 1 cup bacon
- $^1/_2$ red onion
- 1 cup avocado mayo
- 1 cup macadamia nuts
- $^1/_2$ cup Monkfruit sweetener
- 1 tablespoon organic apple cider vinegar

DIRECTIONS

1. **Place Macadamia Nuts in a blender and blend until smooth**
2. **Place all ingredients in a bowl and mix well, pour over Macadamia Nuts mixture and serve**

KETO GREEN SPRING SALAD

Serves: **4**
Prep Time: **10** Minutes

Cook Time: **30** Minutes

Total Time: **40** Minutes

INGREDIENTS

- 2-ounces mixed greens
- 2 tablespoons pine nuts
- 1 tablespoon raspberry vinaigrette

- 1 tablespoon parmesan
- 1 slice bacon
- salt and pepper

DIRECTIONS

1. **Cook bacon until crispy**
2. **Place greens in a bowl with the rest of ingredients**
3. **Top with bacon and serve**

KETO EGG SALAD

Serves: **4**

Prep Time: **10** Minutes

Cook Time: **30** Minutes

Total Time: **40** Minutes

INGREDIENTS

- 6 eggs
- 2 celery stalks
- 2 green onion stalks
- 1 green pepper
- 1 tsp mustard
- 2/3 cup mayonnaise

DIRECTIONS

1. Hard boil eggs and remove to a bowl
2. Chop green pepper, onions and celery
3. In a bowl mix all the ingredients and serve

KETO PEPPERONI SALAD

Serves: **4**

Prep Time: **10** Minutes

Cook Time: **30** Minutes

Total Time: **40** Minutes

INGREDIENTS

- ½ avocado
- 12 slices pepperoni
- 1 oz. Mozzarella pears
- Italian seasoning

DIRECTIONS
1. In a bowl mix all ingredients and serve

KETO CHICKEN SALAD

Serves: **4**

Prep Time: **10** Minutes

Cook Time: **30** Minutes

Total Time: **40** Minutes

INGREDIENTS

- 2 ribs celery
- $^1/_2$ tsp pink Himalayan
- 1 tsp fresh dill
- $^1/_2$ cup pecans
- 1 lb. chicken breast
- $^1/_2$ cup mayo
- 1 tsp mustard

DIRECTIONS

1. Preheat oven to 425 F and bake chicken breast for 15-20 minutes
2. Remove chicken and cut into small pieces
3. In a bowl mix all ingredients and toss until chicken is fully coated
4. When ready, add dill and serve

KETO TUNA SALAD

Serves: **4**

Prep Time: **10** Minutes

Cook Time: **30** Minutes

Total Time: **40** Minutes

INGREDIENTS

- 1 can tuna
- $\frac{1}{2}$ tsp dill
- 1 boiled egg
- 1 slice bacon
- 1 tablespoon mayo
- 1 tablespoon sour cream
- 1 tsp mustard
- 1 tablespoon onion

DIRECTIONS

1. Prepare bacon, onion and boil egg
2. In a bowl place tuna, add egg and onion and the rest of ingredients
3. Top with bacon and serve

<u>**SPINACH SALAD**</u>

Serves: **4**

Prep Time: **10** Minutes

Cook Time: **30** Minutes

Total Time: **40** Minutes

INGREDIENTS

- **2 cups spinach**
- **$^{1}/_{2}$ avocado**
- **1 strawberry**

DRESSING

- **2 slices bacon**
- **1 tablespoon avocado oil**
- **pinch red pepper flakes**
- **1 tsp oregano**
- **$^{1}/_{2}$ tsp garlic powder**
- **$^{1}/_{2}$ tsp salt**
- **half lemon**

DIRECTIONS

1. In a bowl mix all dressing ingredients

2. **In another bowl mix salad ingredients and pour dressing over**

3. **Mix well and serve**

KETO POTOTO SALAD

Serves: *1*

Prep Time: *10* Minutes

Cook Time: *10* Minutes

Total Time: *20* Minutes

INGREDIENTS

- 1 cauliflower
- 1 tablespoon mustard
- 1 tsp celery seeds
- $^1/_2$ tsp salt
- $^1/_2$ cup celery
- 1 tsp dill
- $^1/_2$ cup sour cream
- $^1/_2$ cup mayonnaise
- 2 stalks green onions
- 2 hard boiled eggs
- 1 tablespoon white vinegar

DIRECTIONS

1. In a bowl prepare dressing by whisking together sour cream, celery seed, salt, mayonnaise, vinegar and mustard
2. In another bowl mix salad ingredient, pour dressing and mix well

KETO MONGOLAIN BEEF

Serves: *2*

Prep Time: *10* Minutes

Cook Time: *10* Minutes

Total Time: *20* Minutes

INGREDIENTS

- 1 lb. flat iron steak
- $^{1}/_{2}$ cup coconut oil
- 2 green onions

LOW CARB MONGOLIAN BEEF MARINADE

- $^{1}/_{2}$ cup coconut aminos
- 1 tsp ginger
- 1 clove garlic

DIRECTIONS

1. **Cut the flat iron steak into thin slices**
2. **Add the beef to a ziplock bag and add coconut aminos, garlic and ginger, marinate for 1 hour**

3. Add coconut oil to a wok and cook beef on high heat for 2-3 minutes
4. Add green onions, cook for another 1-2 minutes
5. Remove and serve

<u>**PEPPERONI KETO PIZZA**</u>

Serves: *2*

Prep Time: *10* Minutes

Cook Time: *10* Minutes

Total Time: *20* Minutes

INGREDIENTS

- 1 cauli'flour foods crust
- 2 oz. pepperoni
- $1/2$ cup pizza sauce
- salt
- 2-ounces fresh mozzarella
- $1/2$ cup jalapeno

DIRECTIONS

1. Preheat oven to 375 F and place pizza crust on a vented pizza pan, cook for 8-10 minutes
2. Add mozzarella, sauce, pepperoni and jalapeno
3. Place back in the oven for 5-6 minutes
4. Remove and serve

<u>**QUICK KETO PIZZA**</u>

Serves: *4*

Prep Time: *10* Minutes

Cook Time: *10* Minutes

Total Time: *10* Minutes

INGREDIENTS

PIZZA CRUST
- 2 eggs
- 1 tablespoon parmesan cheese
- 1 tablespoon husk powder
- $^1/_2$ tsp Italian seasoning - salt
- 2 tsp frying oil

TOPPINGS
- 1 oz. mozzarella cheese
- 2 tablespoons. Tomato sauce
- 1 tablespoon chopped basil

DIRECTIONS

1. In a bowl mix all pizza crust ingredients

2. **Spoon the mixture into a pan, cook for 1 minute per side**
3. **Add cheese, tomato sauce and broil for 1-2 minutes until cheese is bubbling**

MUSHROOMS PIZZA

Serves: **2**

Prep Time: **10** Minutes

Cook Time: **15** Minutes

Total Time: **25** Minutes

INGREDIENTS

- $1/4$ cup rao's marinara
- pepperoni
- sliced baby bella mushrooms
- sliced ripe olives
- mozzarella

DIRECTIONS

1. Preheat oven to 375 F
2. Spray a pie plate with a non-stick cooking spray
3. Spread marinara on bottom of pie plate
4. Layer mushrooms, pepperoni, olives and top with mozzarella
5. Bake for 10 minutes and serve

BUFFALO KETO CHICKEN TENDERS

Serves: **2**

Prep Time: **10** Minutes

Cook Time: **30** Minutes

Total Time: **40** Minutes

INGREDIENTS

- 1 lb. chicken breast tenders
- 1 cup almond flour
- 1 egg
- 1 tablespoon heavy whipping cream
- 5 oz. buffalo sauce
- salt

DIRECTIONS

1. Preheat oven to 325 F
2. Season chicken with salt, pepper and almond flour
3. Beat 1 egg with heavy cream
4. Dip each tender in the egg and then into seasoned almond flour
5. Place tenders on a baking sheet and bake for 25 minutes or until crispy

6. Remove and serve

KETO LASAGNA

Serves: **4**

Prep Time: **10** Minutes

Cook Time: **30** Minutes

Total Time: **40** Minutes

INGREDIENTS

- 1 lb. ground beef
- 1 cup sauce
- $^3/_4$ cup mozzarella
- 6 tablespoons ricotta
- salt, onion powder, Italian seasoning

DIRECTIONS

1. **Preheat oven to 350 F, brown beef and season**
2. **Being to layer a deep dish with noodle, ricotta, sauce mix and sprinkle with mozzarella, top with cheese**
3. **Bake for 20-25 minutes**
4. **Remove and serve**

KETO PARMESAN CASSEROLE

Serves: **3**

Prep Time: **10** Minutes

Cook Time: **30** Minutes

Total Time: **40** Minutes

INGREDIENTS

- **2 cups cooked chicken**
- **$^1/_2$ tsp basil**
- **1 slice bacon**
- **$^1/_2$ cup marinara sauce**
- **$^1/_2$ tsp red pepper flakes**
- **$^3/_4$ cup mozzarella cheese**
- **$^1/_2$ cup Parmesan cheese**

DIRECTIONS

1. **Preheat the oven to 325 F**
2. **Lay out the chicken in the pan and spread the marinara sauce all over**
3. **Dredge the top with parmesan, red pepper flakes, mozzarella and sprinkle bacon and basil**
4. **Bake for 20-25 minutes, remove and serve**

<u>**KETO CHEESE MEATBALLS**</u>

Serves: *2*
Prep Time: *10* Minutes

Cook Time: *10* Minutes

Total Time: *20* Minutes

INGREDIENTS

- $^1/_2$ lbs. beef mince
- 2 tablespoons parmesan cheese
- $^1/_2$ tsp salt
- $^1/_2$ tsp pepper
- $^1/_4$ lbs. cheese
- 1 tsp garlic powder

DIRECTIONS

1. **Cut the cheese into cubes**
2. **Mix all dry ingredients with the ground beef**
3. **Wrap the cubes of cheese in mince and pan fry the meatballs**

KETO CHEESY BACON CHICKEN

Serves: **4**

Prep Time: **10** Minutes

Cook Time: **30** Minutes

Total Time: **40** Minutes

INGREDIENTS

- **5 chicken breasts**
- **2 tablespoons seasoning rub**
- **$^1/_2$ lbs. bacon**
- **3 oz. shredded cheddar**
- **barbecue sauce**

DIRECTIONS

1. **Preheat oven to 375 F and spray a baking sheet with cooking spray**
2. **Rub both sides of chicken breast with seasoning rub and top with bacon, bake for 25 minutes**
3. **Remove from oven, sprinkle with cheese and serve**

KETO CHEESEBURGER

Serves: **2**

Prep Time: **10** Minutes

Cook Time: **60** Minutes

Total Time: **70** Minutes

INGREDIENTS

- 2 lbs. ground beef
- 2 eggs
- $^1/_2$ cup grated parmesan
- 1 small onion
- 1 tsp salt
- 1 tsp garlic powder
- $^1/_2$ cup cheddar cheese

DIRECTIONS

1. In a bowl mix all ingredients except cheddar cheese, add the end add cheese cubes
2. Place mixture into a sprayed oven dish and form a meatloaf shape
3. Bake at 325 F for 50 minutes
4. Remove and serve

CAKE

CHEESECAKE KETO FAT BOMBS

Serves: *12*

Prep Time: *10* Minutes

Cook Time: *10* Minutes

Total Time: *20* Minutes

INGREDIENTS

- 5 oz. cream cheese
- 2 oz. frozen strawberries
- 2 oz. butter
- 1 oz. swerve sweetener
- 1 tsp vanilla extract

DIRECTIONS

1. Puree the strawberries using a blender
2. In a bowl mix sweetener, vanilla, pureed strawberries and mix well
3. Microwave cream cheese and combine with the rest of ingredients

4. Add butter to the mixture and mix with an electric mixer

5. Divide into 10-12 round silicone molds and freeze for 1-2 hours before serving

KETO BROWNIES

Serves: **12**
Prep Time: **10** Minutes

Cook Time: **20** Minutes

Total Time: **30** Minutes

INGREDIENTS

- ½ cup almond flour
- ½ tsp baking powder
- 1 tablespoon instant coffee
- 2 oz. chocolate
- 1 egg
- ½ tsp vanilla extract
- ½ cup cacao powder
- 2/3 cup Erythritol
- 8 tablespoons utter

DIRECTIONS

1. Preheat oven to 325 F
2. In a medium bowl whisk almond flour, baking powder, Erythritol, cocoa powder and instant coffee
3. In another bowl melt chocolate and butter and whisk in the eggs and vanilla
4. Add to dry ingredients and mix well
5. Transfer batter into baking dish and bake for 20 minutes

6. Remove and serve

KETO ICE CREAM

Prep Time: **10** Minutes
Cook Time: **20** Minutes
Total Time: **30** Minutes

INGREDIENTS

- 2 cups heavy cream
- 1 tablespoon milk powder
- $^{1}/_{2}$ tsp xanthum gum
- 1 tsp vanilla extract
- 1 cup whole milk
- $^{1}/_{2}$ cup truvia baking blend

DIRECTIONS

1. In a bowl mix milk powder, sweetener, xanthum gum
2. Pour in cream, vanilla extract, milk and mix until sweetener is dissolved
3. Pour into ice cream maker and churn until set
4. Serve when ready

KETO EGG CREPES

Serves: *2*

Prep Time: *10* Minutes

Cook Time: *10* Minutes

Total Time: *20* Minutes

INGREDIENTS

- 5 eggs
- 5 oz. cream cheese
- 1 tsp cinnamon
- 1 tablespoon sugar substitute
- butter

FILLING

- 7 tablespoons butter
- $1/2$ cup sugar substitute
- 1 tablespoon cinnamon

DIRECTIONS

1. Blend all of the crepe ingredients until smooth
2. Pour batter into the pan and cook 1-2 minutes per side
3. Remove and pour mixture over the crepes
   4. For crepes mixture mix cinnamon and sweetener in a bowl
5. Serve when ready

KETO NAAN

Serves: *4*
Prep Time: *10* Minutes
Cook Time: **30** Minutes
Total Time: **40** Minutes

INGREDIENTS

- $^1/_2$ cup coconut flour
- 1 tablespoon psyllium husk
- 1 tablespoon ghee
- $^1/_2$ tsp baking powder
- $^1/_2$ tsp salt
- 1 cup boiling water

DIRECTIONS

1. In a bowl mix all ingredients and refrigerate
2. Divine the dough into 6 balls
3. Heat a cast iron skillet over medium heat and place ice naan ball
4. Cook for 2-3 minutes remove and serve

PEANUT BUTTER COOKIES

Prep Time: **10** Minutes

Cook Time: **30** Minutes

Total Time: **40** Minutes

INGREDIENTS

- 1 cup peanut butter
- 1 tsp vanilla
- 1 tsp baking powder
- $\frac{1}{2}$ tsp salt
- $\frac{1}{2}$ cup keto sweetener
- 1 egg

DIRECTIONS

1. **Preheat oven to 325 F**
2. **Cream together all ingredients**
3. **Refrigerate for 15-20 minutes**
4. **Roll dough into balls and place on a parchment paper**
5. **Bake for 12-15 minutes**

BUTTERY KETO CREPES

Serves: **2**

Prep Time: **10** Minutes

Cook Time: **10** Minutes

Total Time: **20** Minutes

INGREDIENTS

- **3 eggs**
- **$^1/_2$ tsp vanilla extract**
- **$^1/_2$ tsp cinnamon**
- **3 oz. cream cheese**
- **2 tsp sweetener**
- **2 tablespoons butter**

DIRECTIONS

1. **In a blender place all the ingredients and blend until smooth**
2. **In a skillet pour batter and cook each crepe for 1-2 minutes per side or until ready**
3. **Remove and serve with berries, maple syrup or jam**

KETO LEMON FAT BOMB

Serves: **4**

Prep Time: **10** Minutes

Cook Time: **10** Minutes

Total Time: **20** Minutes

INGREDIENTS

- $^1/_2$ cup coconut oil
- 3 tablespoons butter
- 3 oz. cream cheese
- 2 tsp lemon juice
- 2 tsp sugar substitute

DIRECTIONS

1. **Place all ingredients in a mixing bowl and mix thoroughly**
2. **Spoon 2 tablespoons into cupcake holders and freeze**
3. **Remove and serve**

PEANUT BUTTER BALLS

Prep Time: **10** Minutes

Cook Time: **30** Minutes

Total Time: **40** Minutes

INGREDIENTS

- 1 cup peanuts finely chopped
- 1 cup peanut butter
- 1 cup powdered sweetener

- 6 oz. sugar free chocolate chips

DIRECTIONS

1. In a bowl mix peanut butter, sweetener, chopped peanuts, divide dough into 12 pieces and shape into balls and place on a wax paper
2. Melt chocolate and dip each peanut butter ball in the chocolate and place back on the wax paper

Refrigerate and serve

NUT FREE KETO BROWNIE

Serves: **8**

Prep Time: **10** Minutes

Cook Time: **20** Minutes

Total Time: **30** Minutes

INGREDIENTS

- 5 eggs
- $^1/_4$ lb. butter
- 2 oz. cocoa
- $^1/_2$ tsp baking powder
- 2 tsp vanilla
- $^1/_4$ lb. cream cheese
- 3 tablespoons sweetener of choice

DIRECTIONS

1. **Place all the ingredients in a lender and blend until smooth**
2. **Pour mixture into a baking dish**
3. **Bake at 325 F for 20 minutes**
4. **Remove slice into squares and serve**

<u>COFFEE SMOOTHIE</u>

Serves: **1**

Prep Time: **5** Minutes

Cook Time: **5** Minutes

Total Time: **10** Minutes

INGREDIENTS

- 5 oz. cold coffee
- 3 oz. heavy cream
- 3 oz. almond milk
- 1 oz. sugar free chocolate syrup
- 1 oz. caramel syrup
- 1 tablespoon cocoa
- 12 oz. ice

DIRECTIONS

1. In a blender place all the ingredients and blend until smooth
2. Pour in a glass and serve

CHAI PUMPKIN SMOOTHIE

Serves: **1**

Prep Time: **5** Minutes

Cook Time: **5** Minutes

Total Time: **10** Minutes

INGREDIENTS

- $^3/_4$ **cup coconut milk**
- **2 tablespoon pumpkin puree**
- **1 tablespoon MCT oil**
- **1 tsp chai tea**
- **1 tsp alcohol free vanilla**
- $^1/_2$ **tsp pumpkin pie spice**
- $^1/_2$ **frozen avocado**

DIRECTIONS

1. **In a blender place all the ingredients and blend until smooth**
2. **Pour in a glass and serve**

<u>**CASHEW SMOOTHIE**</u>

Serves: **1**
Prep Time: **5** Minutes

Cook Time: **5** Minutes

Total Time: **10** Minutes

INGREDIENTS

- **1 cup cashew mik**
- **1 tablespoon keto MCT oil**
- **1 tablespoon keto nut butter**
- **1 tsp maca powder**
- **1 handful ice**

DIRECTIONS

1. **In a blender place all the ingredients and blend until smooth**
2. **Pour in a glass and serve**

BREAKFAST SMOOTHIE

Prep Time: **5** Minutes
Cook Time: **5** Minutes
Total Time: **10** Minutes

INGREDIENTS

- $1/_2$ cup almond milk
- $1/_2$ cup coconut milk
- $1/_2$ coconut yoghurt
- $1/_2$ tsp stevia
- 3 strawberries

DIRECTIONS

1. **In a blender place all the ingredients and blend until smooth**
2. **Pour in a glass and serve**

KETO MILKSHAKE SMOOTHIE

Serves: **1**
Prep Time: **5** Minutes
Cook Time: **5** Minutes
Total Time: **10** Minutes

INGREDIENTS

- **6 oz. plain almond milk**
- **3 oz. crushed ice**
- **1 oz. heavy whipping cream**
- **1 oz. raspberries**
- **$^3/_4$ oz. sweetener of choice**
- **$^1/_2$ oz. cream cheese**

DIRECTIONS

1. **In a blender place all the ingredients and blend until smooth**
2. **Pour in a glass and serve**

AVOCADO SMOOTHIE

Serves: **1**

Prep Time: **5** Minutes

Cook Time: **5** Minutes

Total Time: **10** Minutes

INGREDIENTS

- $^1/_2$ avocado
- 2 tablespoons cocoa powder
- 2/3 cup coconut milk
- $^1/_2$ cup crushed ice
- $^1/_2$ cup water
- pinch of salt
- 1 tsp lime juice
- stevia

DIRECTIONS

1. **In a blender place all the ingredients and blend until smooth**
2. **Pour in a glass and serve**

COLLAGEN SMOOTHIE

Serves: **1**

Prep Time: **5** Minutes

Cook Time: **5** Minutes

Total Time: **10** Minutes

INGREDIENTS

- 4 ice cubes
- $^1/_2$ avocado

- 1 scoop keto chocolate collagen
- 1 tablespoon chia seeds
- 1 tablespoon almond butter
- $^3/_4$ cup heavy whipping cream
- 1 cup water

DIRECTIONS

1. In a blender place all the ingredients and blend until smooth
2. Pour in a glass and serve

FAT BOMB SMOOTHIE

Serves: **1**

Prep Time: **5** Minutes

Cook Time: **5** Minutes

Total Time: **10** Minutes

INGREDIENTS

- 2.5 oz avocado
- 1 scoop collagen
- 1 tablespoon cacao powder
- 1 cup almond milk
- 1 cup ice

DIRECTIONS

1. **In a blender place all the ingredients and blend until smooth**
2. **Pour in a glass and serve**

CINNAMON SMOOTHIE

Serves: **1**
Prep Time: **5** Minutes
Cook Time: **5** Minutes
Total Time: **10** Minutes

INGREDIENTS

- $^1/_2$ cup coconut milk
- $^1/_2$ cup water
- 2 ice cubes
- 1 tablespoon coconut oil
- $^1/_2$ tsp cinnamon
- 1 tablespoon chia seeds
- $^1/_2$ cup vanilla protein powder

DIRECTIONS

1. **In a blender place all the ingredients and blend until smooth**
2. **Pour in a glass and serve**

TROPICAL SMOOTHIE

Serves: **1**
Prep Time: **5** Minutes
Cook Time: **5** Minutes
Total Time: **10** Minutes

- ¹/₂ tsp banana extract
- ¹/₂ tsp blueberry extract
- ¹/₂ tsp mango extract
- stevia
- 1 tablespoon oil
- ¹/₂ cup sour cream
- ice cubes
- ³/₄ cup coconut milk

DIRECTIONS
1. **In a blender place all the ingredients and blend until smooth**
2. **Pour in a glass and serve**

What is the Paleo Diet?

For 2.5 million years, early man foraged and hunted for seafood, meat, vegetables,
fruit, nuts, roots and seeds. This period of time before the development of agriculture
is
known as the Paleolithic era. The Paleo diet is also known as the Stone Age diet,
hunter-gathering diet and the caveman diet. No matter what you call our ancestors,
some things haven't changed. Man's digestive systems have evolved only the slightest
amount in the 10,000 years since farming changed our diets. Shortened to Paleo, the
modern diet is an approach to nutrition that mimics the early man's diet for ultimate
health.

Our minds are modern, but our bodies and brains still need the same food.
Gastroenterologist Walter L. Voegtlin first popularized the Paleo diet in the 1970's.
He argued in, "The Stone Age Diet," humans as carnivores, chiefly needs fats,
proteins and a small amount of carbohydrates for optimum performance. For the last
30 years, obesity has been increasing in the United States. Our modern diets are
laden with preservatives, processed sugars, and fried foods. Today's health crisis
has led to a renewed interest in Voegtlin's tested approach to healthy living.

Benefits of the Paleo Diet

The advantages of the Paleo Diet have been researched and proven in numerous academic journals. It is amazing how changing what we put in our mouths can cause dramatic changes in our quality of life.

- o <u>Lose fat-</u> Though the Paleo diet is designed as a weight loss plan people inherently lose weight. The foods that make up the Paleo diet are what we call fat burning foods. In fact, the Paleo diet allows you to eat large quantities of delicious food while restricting calories. The result is a lean, fit body.

- o <u>Fight Disease-</u> The Paleo diet is proven to help prevent diabetes, Parkinson's avoid Parkinson's, cancer, heart disease and strokes.

- o <u>Improve Digestion-</u> Many digestive problems such as, irritable bowel syndrome, Crohn's disease and indigestion can be avoided.

- o <u>Combats Acne–</u> Eating the Paleo way means avoiding the foods that cause acne. When sebum is overproduced or obstructed the sebaceous glands enlarge and form pimples. Foods in the Paleo diet do not cause the insulin spikes that cause a sebum boost. As a result, you can expect smoother, more attractive skin.

- o <u>Feel Good-</u> Not only does the Paleo diet help people healthier and look younger it also makes you feel better. Paleo supporters swear by the caveman lifestyle because it just "feels" right. The only way to find out the energy and confidence they experience is to try it for yourself.

Diet Basics

People assume the Paleo Diet is complicated are difficult to follow. It is actually quite simple. Eat real foods. For a guideline on portions, 56–65%

of your calories should come from animals, 36–45% from plant based foods. Keep proteins high at 19-35% carbohydrates at 22-40% and fat at 28-58%.

What to Eat

Eating a Paleo Diet is more about experimenting than limitations. Mother Nature provides a large variety of delicious foods to explore. Instead of settling for a box of processed macaroni and cheese, feast on a meal that excites your taste buds and your energy level. Here is a small list of the many foods to incorporate into your diet.

PROTIENS

Meat	Gam	Poult	Fish	Shel	Eggs
Beef	Pheas	Goos	Tun	Lobst	Chicke
Veal	Deer	Chick	Salm	Shri	Goose
Pork	Duck	Turke	Trou	Scall	Duck
Lamb	Wild	Quail	Hali	Crab	Quail
Goat	Rabbi	Duck	Sole	Clam	

Rabbit	Moose	Bass	Mussels
Sheep	Woodcock	Haddock	Oysters
Wild Boar	Elk	Turbot	
Bison		Cod	
		Tilapia	
		Walleye	
		Flatfish	
		Grouper	
		Mackerel	
		Herring	
		Anchovy	

VEGETABLES

Standards	Green Leafy	Squash	Root	Mushrooms
Cauliflower	Collard	Butternut	Turnips	Oyster
Broccoli	Lettuce	Spaghetti	Carrots	Button
Celery	Spinach	Acorn	Beets	Portabella
Bell Peppers	Watercress	Pumpkin	Parsnips	Chanterelle
Onions	Beet Top	Zucchini	Artichokes	Porcini
Leeks	Dandelion	Yellow	Rutabaga	Shiitake
Green Onions	Swiss Chard	Buttercup	Sweet	Crimini
Eggplant	Mustard	Crookneck	Radish	Morel
Brussels	Kale		Yams	
Artichokes	Turnip Greens		Cassava	
Asparagus	Seaweed			
Cucumber	Endive			
Cabbage	Arugula			
Okra				
Avocados				

SUPPORTING PLAYERS

Fats	Fruits	Nuts & Seeds	Flavor Enhancers	Fresh & Dry Herbs
Olive Oil	Apples	Brazil Nuts	Cayenne Pepper	Parsley
Avocado	Oranges	Pistachios	Chilies	Thyme
Coconut Oil	Bananas	Sunflower Seeds	Ginger	Lavender
Clarified Butter	Strawberry	Pumpkin Seeds	Onions	Mint
Lard	Cranberry	Sesame Seeds	Garlic	Rosemary
Tallow	Grapefruit	Pecans	Black Pepper	Chives
Veal Fat	Peaches	Walnuts	Hot Peppers	Tarragon
Duck Fat	Pears	Macadamia Nuts	Star Anise	Oregano
Coconut Flesh	Nectarines	Pine Nuts	Mustard Seeds	Dill
Nut Oils	Plums	Chestnuts	Fennel Seeds	Bay Leaves
Nut Butter	Pomegranates	Cashews	Cumin	Sage
Lamb Fat	Pineapple	Hazelnuts	Turmeric	Coriander
	Grapes	Almonds	Cinnamon	
	Papaya		Paprika	
	Cantaloupe		Nutmeg	
	Kiwi		Cloves	
	Lychee		Vanilla	

Foods to Eliminate

The main foods to eliminate are processed foods, the largest source of toxicity and malnutrition. Processed foods are the easiest items to eat these days, and we eat entirely too much. Grains that form the base of sandwich breads, cereals and pasta have no place in the Paleo Diet. Also, the processed fats and vegetable seed oils are also counterproductive to our health. Legumes, especially soy, and vegetable seed oils should be banished from your diet. There are no refined sugars little dairy and absolutely no processed foods in the Paleo plan.

Tips for the Paleo Lifestyle

Unfortunately, the cheapest and quickest foods available today are usually the least nutritious. Our busy lifestyles have our kids raised on a diet of processed and fast foods. The popular culture even makes eating real foods an odd concept. Even knowing the proven benefits, some never try the Paleo diet because they believe it is too difficult. Living a long, healthy fulfilling life is well worth a few small changes. While not as easy as stopping at a drive through, maintaining a Paleo lifestyle is realistic with a few tips.

Stay Organized- The number one tip is to be organized and prepared. The biggest challenge will be to have Paleo foods available at your home and plan your meals. You are much more likely to eat healthy food choices if it is readily available at home.

- Change How You Shop- Find the best farmers markets, butchers and grocery stores in your area. Before going to the grocery have a list of items you plan to pick up. Also, shop the perimeter of grocery stores to avoid the aisles filled with processed foods. This may be difficult at first, but after a month or so you will know longer feel a need to peruse the sugar aisles.

- Clean Your Pantry- Clear your cupboards of all the cereals, pasta, and processed foods in your cabinets. Don't worry. You will replace these foods with much more satisfying fresh and healthy foods.

- Learn to Work the Kitchen- Unlike a diet based on grains, there are many foods to eat on the Paleo Diet you should never become bored. The best way to take advantage of everything nature has to offer is to learn how to cook. By combining the diverse flavors, there is an endless amount of tasty dishes to excite your taste buds.

- <u>Dress Your Food-</u> Most of the condiments on the store shelves are filled with preservatives. However, you can enhance the flavor of your foods by making your own condiments at home. Ketchup, mustard, salad dressings and sauces can be made at home naturally with delicious results.

- <u>Exercise-</u> Just changing your eating habits will cause you to lose weight naturally on the Paleo Diet. Add exercise to the mix, and you will be amazed at how quickly you notice a difference. Your true, toned physique will come out as pounds shed. You will also notice the amount of energy increased compared to when you ate a traditional diet. Start feeling strong, energetic, mentally sharper and all around younger.

- <u>Join Support System-</u> Find chat rooms and forums where like-minded people meet. Participate at a gym where the Paleo Diet is the main lifestyle choice. It is nice to share ideas on the best Paleo books, and even give advice on keeping true to the diet plan. Joining a community online or in person is extremely motivating

  when you learn about how the other member's lives improved just from staying true to the Paleo way.

Paleo Friendly Desserts

One of the biggest stumbling blocks with the Paleo Diet plan is desserts. Most desserts have unnatural sweeteners and starchy carbs that spike insulin levels. Most sweet treats are a recipe for disaster. However, with kids, special celebrations and Birthdays sometimes a sweet treat is in order. There are some very tasty Paleo desserts that can help you transition fully into the Paleo lifestyle without indulging in bad choices or having a gluten stomachache. While it is not a good idea to eat desserts after every meal, Paleo friendly desserts can stop hardcore cravings from your pre-Paleo days.

Here is a list of whole food substitutions you can use to whip delicious Paleo friendly desserts together.

- Almond flour- Grinding almonds create nutritious, high protein flour perfect for making muffins breads and of course, traditional macaroons.

- Raw Honey– Because honey can be eaten straight from the tree, it is considered a true Paleo sweetener. Though it is a whole food, honey is highly caloric and does spike the insulin level, so leave sparingly. However, honey is the perfect sugar substitute.

- Cocoa- Unsweetened dark chocolate has nutritious antioxidants and sticks to the limited dairy rules. Opt for the natural cocoa over the Dutch processed version that loses its benefits during processing.

- Pure Vanilla Extract– Pure vanilla extract is a staple in any bakers cupboard. Just make sure to buy the pure stuff not the cheap flavoring.

Coconut Oil- Coconut oil is a medium chain fatty acid, which means it transfers directly to the liver where it is used for energy instead of being stored directly as fat. It also stimulates the thyroid gland helping speed up metabolism. Coconut oil adds a subtle sweetness to cobblers pancakes and other baked recipes.

- Coconut Milk- A great dairy substitute, coconut milk contains lauric acid. Lauric acid is proven to fight influenza, herpes, HIV as well as improve the immune system. Use coconut oil to make ice cream, hot cocoa, pudding, and even egg nog.

- Nuts– Nuts are loaded with good fats the bodies need. Hazelnuts, pecans, macademians and almonds are lifesavers in the kitchen. Use nuts for pie crusts, candies or even as simple spiced nut blend.

- Frozen Fruit- Freeze berries to make easy desserts. Use them to make rich frothy smoothies or sorbet. Frozen grapes and cherries taste delicious straight from the freezer. Try frozen bananas on a stick or blended down for a creamy ice cream experience.

- Dates- Dates are natural sweeteners that do not add its own flavor like honey. They contain simple sugars like dextrose and fructose that are easy to digest and replenish your energy. Blend dates in the food processor with wet ingredients when baking. They also work well for binding snack bars.

CONCLUSION

The Paleo Diet is proven to shed pounds and have a healthier life. Add exercise to the mix and you can achieve the lean, sexy bodies seen on fitness models. Despite popular belief, the Paleo lifestyle is not restrictive and can actually open your palette to a whole new world of culinary experiences. There are a variety of high quality cookbooks and website that will help you along the way. Once you experience the transformation you will wonder how you ever functioned. Get the most of your life and enjoy optimum fitness with the Paleo diet plan.

Paleo Diet
Recipes

Fresh herb meatballs

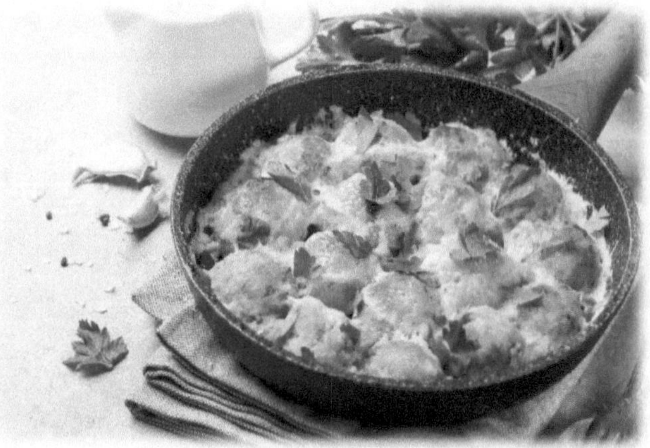

Serve these with a marinara or spaghetti sauce and over spaghetti squash or zucchini noodles if desired.

INGREDIENTS

- 1 lb ground beef;
- 1 lb ground pork;
- $1/2$ onion, minced;
- $1/2$ cup fresh basil, finely minced;
- $1/2$ cup fresh parsley, finely minced;
- 1 cup spinach, finely minced;
- 4 eggs;
- $1/2$ cup almond meal;
- 1 tbsp dried oregano;
- 4 cloves garlic, minced;
- Sea salt and freshly ground black pepper to taste;

PREPARATION

1 Preheat your oven to 350 F.

2 Combine all the ingredients in a bowl and mix well with your hands to combine. You can use a food processor to reduce the basil, parsley and spinach to a finer mixture before adding it to the ground meat. Season the mixture to taste with sea salt and freshly ground black pepper.

3 Make small balls the size of a golf ball and place them apart on a baking sheet, then place them in the preheated oven to cook for about 25 minutes, until well cooked.

Citrus pork rib roast

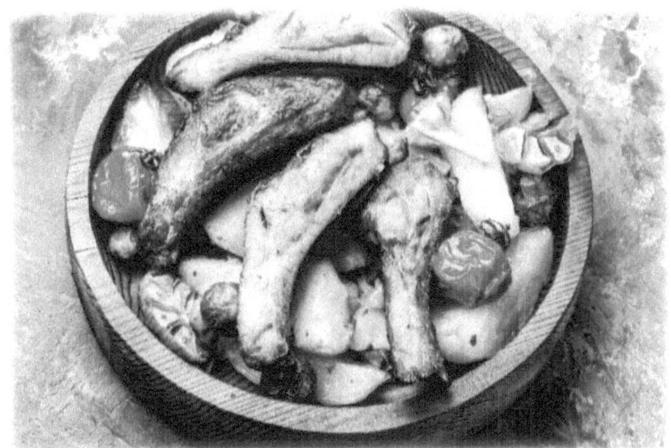

Serve these with roasted or steamed vegetables. Alternatively, this roast is also great with apples or pears roasted for about 1 hour at 350 F.

INGREDIENTS

- 1 pork rib roast, about 4 lbs;
- 3 cloves garlic;
- 3 cloves;
- Juice and zest of 2 lemons;
- Juice and zest of 2 oranges;
- 10 bay leaves;
- 4 rosemary sprigs;
- 1 tbsp fennel seeds, chopped;
- $1/2$ tbsp Juniper berries, crushed with the side of a knife;
- 2 tbsp extra-virgin olive oil;
- Cooking fat, melted;
- Sea salt and freshly ground black pepper to taste;

PREPARATION

1 Make small incisions on the fatty side of the pork roast and insert a garlic clove and a clove in
each
of them.

2 Combine the olive oil, 2 tablespoons cooking fat, and the juice and zest of the lemons and oranges in a baking dish together with the bay leaves, rosemary, fennel seeds and Juniper berries.

3 Season to taste with sea salt and black pepper and place the roast in the marinade and in the refrigerator to marinate overnight.

4 Get the roast out of the refrigerator before cook- ing so it tempers to room temperature.

5 Preheat your oven to 350 F.

6 Scrape the marinade off the roast and brown it all over in a skillet set over a medium heat.

7 Place back the roast in a clean baking dish and roast for about 1 $^1/_2$ hours, until an instant read thermometer indicates 145 F in the thickest part.

8 Let the roast rest for about 15 minutes before carving and serving.

Crock pot cabbage rolls

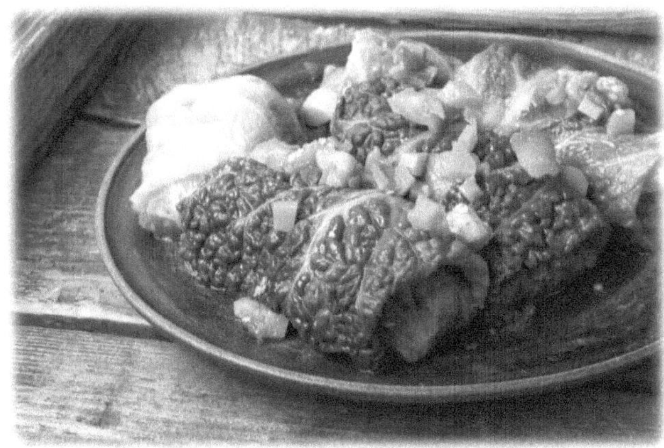

INGREDIENTS

- 12 large cabbage leaves;
- 1 egg;
- $^1/_4$ cup chicken or beef stock;
- $^1/_4$ cup chopped onion;
- 1 lb ground beef;
- 1 cup cauliflower, grated;
- 1 can (8 oz.) tomato sauce;
- 1 tbsp lemon juice;
- Sea salt and freshly ground black pepper to taste;

PREPARATION

1 Blanch the cabbage leaves by placing them in a pot of boiling salted water for about 2 minutes, until the cabbage leaves start to soften. Drain and run under cold water to stop the cooking.

2 Combine together in a bowl the stock, onion, ground beef, cauliflower and egg. Season the mixture to taste with sea salt and freshly ground black pepper.

3 Place the soft cabbage leaves on a flat surface and fill each one with 1/12 of the meat mixture near the base of the leaves.

4 Fold the sides of the leaves and roll them on themselves to close up the mixture inside.

5 Prepare the sauce by combining together the tomato sauce with the lemon juice. Season the sauce to taste with sea salt and freshly ground black pepper.

6 Place the stuffed cabbage rolls inside a crock pot and pour the tomato sauce over.

7 Cook on Low for 7 to 9 hours.

Mushroom and Hazelnut chicken

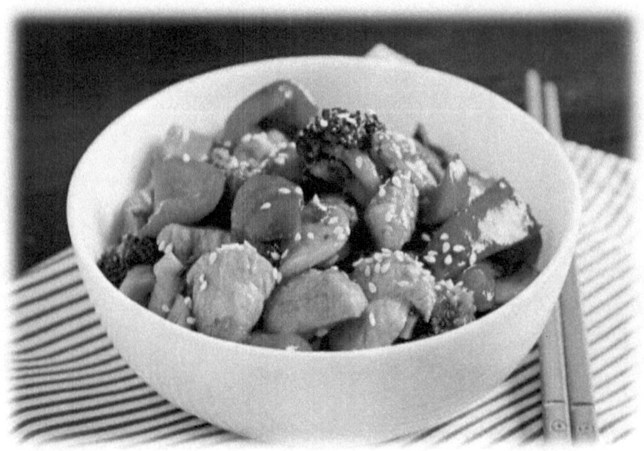

INGREDIENTS

- 4 boneless chicken breasts;
- $\frac{1}{2}$ lb mushrooms, your favorite kind, finely chopped;
- 1 onion, finely chopped;
- 4 garlic cloves, minced;
- $\frac{1}{4}$ cup hazelnuts, roughly chopped;
- $\frac{1}{2}$ cup chicken stock;
- $\frac{1}{4}$ cup homemade or Dijon mustard;
- 2 tbsp chopped fresh sage;
- Cooking fat;
- Sea salt and freshly ground black pepper to taste;

PREPARATION

1 Preheat your oven to 400 F.

2 Heat some cooking fat in a pan and cook the on- ion with the garlic until the onion is soft, about 7 minutes.

3 Add the mushrooms and cook on a medium heat until all the moisture has evaporated.

4 Set the cooked onion and mushrooms aside in a bowl.

5 Cut the thickest part of each chicken breast with a sharp knife to form a cavity for the stuffing.

6 Stuff each breast with the mushroom and onion stuffing.

7 Secure the breasts with butcher's twine.

8 Add some more cooking fat in the pan you used to cook the stuffing and brown the chicken breasts on each side.

9 Place on a baking sheet in the preheated oven for 15 to 20 minutes, until well cooked.

10 Remove from the oven and let rest while you prepare the gravy.

11 In the same pan you used previously, heat up the stock with the mustard and sage, bring to a simmer and let simmer a few minutes to reduce and thicken to the desired consistency.

12 Cut the twine off the chicken breasts and serve topped off with the pan gravy.

Roast leg of lamb with rosemary & garlic

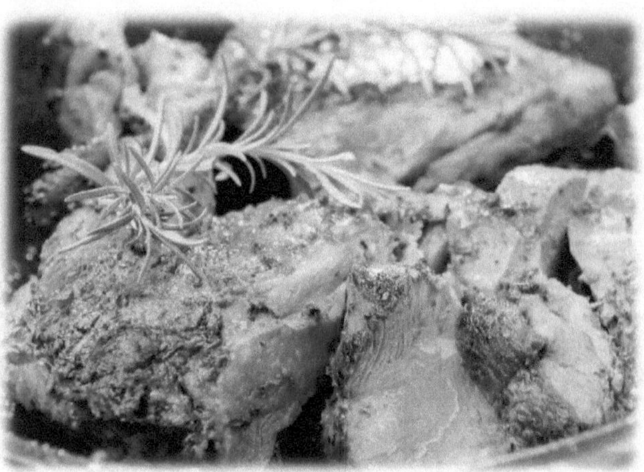

INGREDIENTS

- 1 leg of lamb, bone-in, about 5 $\frac{1}{2}$ lb;
- 12 sprigs rosemary, each sprig cut in half;
- 6 garlic cloves halved lengthwise;
- Cooking fat;
- Sea salt and freshly ground black pepper;

PREPARATION

1 Preheat your oven to 425 F.

2 Refer to the cooking times and temperatures charts to calculate the needed cooking time of the roast depending on its weight and desired doneness.

3 Make 12 incisions on the fatty side of the roast with a sharp knife and insert half a garlic clove and half a rosemary sprig in each incisions.

4 Rub the roast with melted cooking fat of your choice.

5 Place the roast in a roasting pan and roast for a first 15 minutes.

6 Reduce the temperature to 350 F and continue roasting for the remaining of the time, basting with the fat occasionally.

7 When cooked, remove the roast from the oven, place on a cutting board and let rest, covered with foil, for about 20 minutes,.

8 Carve the roast and serve while hot.

Pan-fried Moroccan chicken

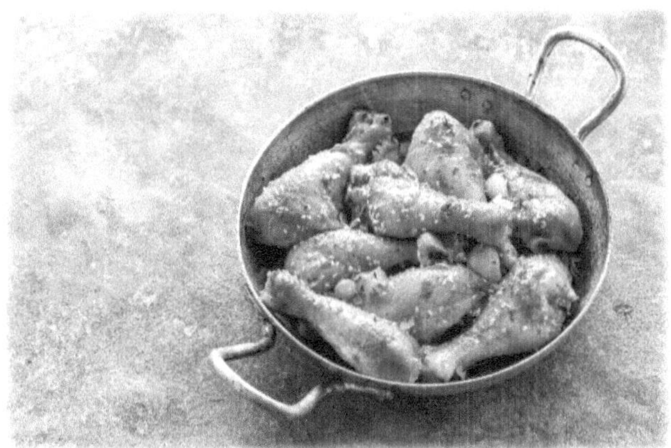

INGREDIENTS

- 1 chilli, seeded and finely chopped;
- 1 tsp chilli flakes;
- 2 garlic cloves, minced;
- Juice of 1 lemon;
- 2 tsp ground cinnamon;
- 3 tsp ground cumin;
- 4 tbsp raisins (optional);
- 4 tbsp pine nuts;
- 1 tbsp olive oil
- Cooking fat;
- 2 lbs chicken fillets, cut into strips;
- 1 orange, halved and sliced;
- 4 tbsp fresh mint, chopped;

PREPARATION

1 Combine the olive oil with the chilli flakes, chopped chilli, garlic, lemon juice, cinnamon,
cumin, pine nuts and raisins, if using. Season to taste with sea salt and freshly ground black pepper.

2 Coat the chicken strips in the rub and place in the refrigerator to marinate for 30 minutes.

3 Heat some cooking fat in a large frying pan and cook the marinated chicken strips on a medium heat for about 2 minutes.

4 Flip the chicken strips over, add the orange slices and cook for a further 2 or 3 minutes, until well cooked.

5 Stir in the fresh mint and serve.

Beef, cabbage and mushroom crock pot stew

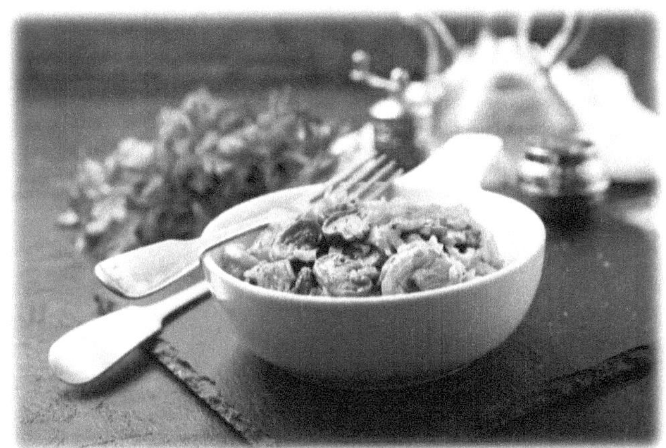

INGREDIENTS

- 3 lbs beef chuck, cut into 1-inch cubes;
- 1 medium onion, chopped;
- 6 fresh shitake mushrooms;
- 3 garlic cloves;
- 1 can (14 oz.) chopped tomatoes or 3 fresh tomatoes, chopped;
- 5 carrots, cut into 1-inch pieces;
- 3 cups beef or chicken stock;
- 1 head cabbage, coarsely chopped;
- Cooking fat;
- Sea salt and freshly ground black pepper to taste;

PREPARATION

1 Season the beef cubes to taste with sea salt and freshly ground black pepper;

2 Using a pot, brown the meat on all sides in some cooking fat over a medium heat.

3 Set the beef cubes aside, add some cooking fat if needed and cook the onions with the mush-rooms until soft, about 5 minutes.

4 Season to taste with sea salt and freshly ground black pepper, add the garlic and cook for anoth-er minute or two.

5 Place the cooked onions and mushrooms with the beef in your crock pot with the wine, carrots, stock, tomatoes and season again to taste.

6 Cook on Low for about 6 hours.

7 Add the chopped cabbage and cook for another hour.

8 Adjust the seasoning if needed and serve.

Coconut red snapper and pineapple salsa

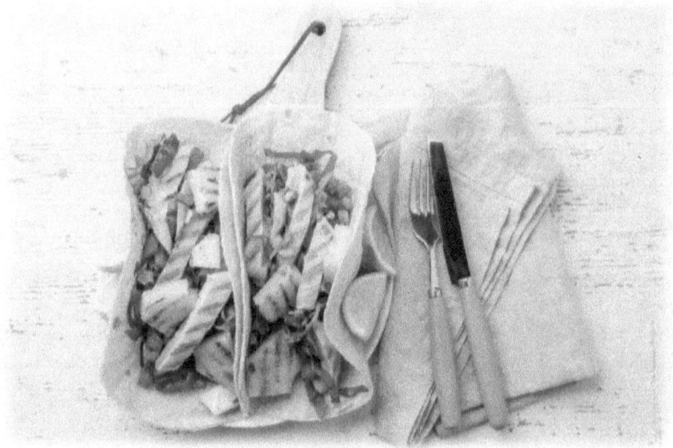

Salsa
INGREDIENTS
PREPARATION

1 Combine the juice of 2 limes with the garlic in a bowl.

- 1 small pineapple, diced;
- 1 onion, finely diced;
- 1 bell pepper, finely diced;
- 1 tsp paprika;
- 1 tsp lemon juice;
- 2 tsp extra-virgin olive oil;
- Sea salt and freshly ground black pepper to taste;

Fish
- 4 red snapper fillets;
- Juice of 2 $\frac{1}{2}$ limes;
- 1 clove garlic, minced;
- 4 tbsp coconut flakes;
- 2 tsp fresh thyme leaves;
- Cooking fat;
- Sea salt and freshly ground black pepper to taste;

2 Place the fish fillets in a baking dish and pour the marinade over them. Let marinate
at room

temperature for 1 to 2 hours.

3 Place the thyme leaves in a bowl with the co- conut flakes and coat the snapper fillets in that mixture, pressing them so the coconut sticks.

4 Combine the pineapple in a bowl together with the onion, bell pepper, paprika, olive oil and lemon juice. Season to taste with sea salt and freshly ground black pepper.

5 Heat a large skillet over a medium heat and cook the fillets in some cooking fat for about 3 to 4 minutes per side, until nice and crispy on the outside. Add the remaining lime juice in the last minute of cooking along with another 1 tbsp cooking fat.

6 Serve with the prepared pineapple salsa on the side.

Omelet with sausage crust

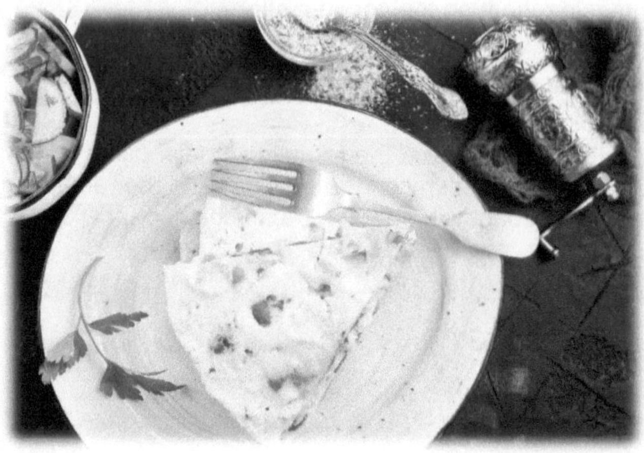

This is a nice and bulky pie where the crust is made out of sausage and the filling is an omelet with
bell pep- pers and onions. This one is bound to become a favorite.
Crust

INGREDIENTS
PREPARATION

1 Preheat your oven to 350 F.

* $3/4$ lb ground beef;

* $3/4$ lb breakfast sausage;

* 2 eggs, lightly beaten;

* $1/2$ cup onion, minced;

* $1/4$ cup chopped basil;

* $3/4$ tsp oregano;

* Sea salt and freshly ground black pepper to taste;
Omelet

* 6 eggs;

* 2 tbsp coconut milk;

* $1/4$ tsp onion powder;

* 1/8 cup red bell pepper, chopped;

* 2 tbsp chives, chopped;

2 Combine together in a bowl the ground beef, sausage meat, eggs, onion, basil (keep 1 tbsp of the basil for the omelet filling), oregano and season to taste. Set 1 cup of the mixture aside.

3 Line the rest of the mixture in a round 10-inch pie plate as you would a normal

crust by press-ing everything together firmly.

4 Bake the crust for 15 minutes in the preheated oven.

5 Meanwhile, sauté the reserved meat mixture in a bit of cooking fat until well cooked. Let cool.

6 Remove the pre-baked crust from the oven and set aside to cool for about 10 minutes.

7 Combine the eggs, coconut milk, onion powder and red bell peppers in a bowl with a whisk. Season to taste with sea salt and freshly ground black pepper.
8 Pour the egg mixture over the cooled sausage crust and then sprinkle the remaining 1 cup basil and sausage mixture as well as the chopped chives and bake in the preheated oven for 30 minutes

Brussel sprout and bacon medley

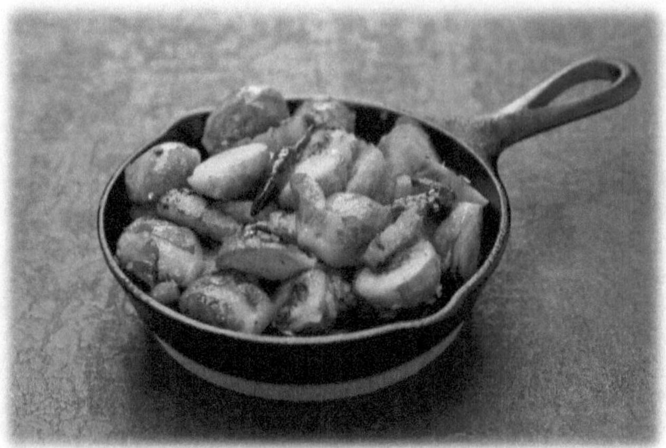

This is a great side to serve with baked or pan fried fish.

INGREDIENTS

- 5 slices bacon;
- 1 onion, chopped;
- 1 $\frac{1}{2}$ lbs Brussel sprouts;
- 1 cup chicken stock;
- Freshly ground black pepper to taste;

PREPARATION

1 Heat a skillet over a medium heat and cook the bacon until crispy, about 7 minutes on each side.

2 Pat the cooked bacon dry and cut it into $\frac{1}{4}$-inch pieces.

3 Cook the chopped onion in the rendered fat in the skillet you used for the bacon for about 2 minutes.

4 Add the whole Brussel sprouts, stir well and cook for another 3 minutes, until they start to soften.

5 Pour in the chicken stock, bring to a boil and then reduce to a simmer and simmer for 10 min-utes, covered.

6 When cooked, drain the liquid and place the Brussel sprouts in a serving dish sprinkled with the cooked bacon.

German pork hocks

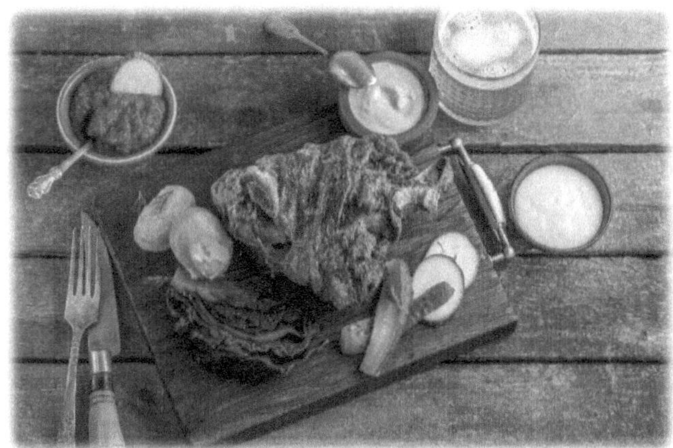

In Germany those pork hocks are often served with sauerkraut. Feel free though to enjoy those with any of your favorite sides. Pork hocks are a nice and cheap cut of meat that offers a delicious taste when cooked gently and slowly.

INGREDIENTS

- 1 leek, cleaned thoroughly and cut into 1-inch pieces;
- 2 celery stalks, diced;
- 1 carrot, diced;
- 1 onion, diced;
- 2 pork hocks;
- Sea salt to taste;
- 1 tsp whole black peppercorns;

PREPARATION

1 Place the hocks in a large pot with the leeks, cel- ery, onion, carrot and whole peppercorns. Add some sea salt to taste.

2 Fill the pot with water to cover the hocks and vegetables, bring to a boil and then reduce to a simmer and let simmer for 2 to 3 hours, until the meat is very tender.

3 Drain, reserve the liquid and preheat your oven to 425 F.

4 Place the cooked hocks with the vegetables in a baking dish with some of the reserved cooking liquid.

5 Place in the oven to roast for about 30 minutes, basting it from time to time.

Sweet potato chips

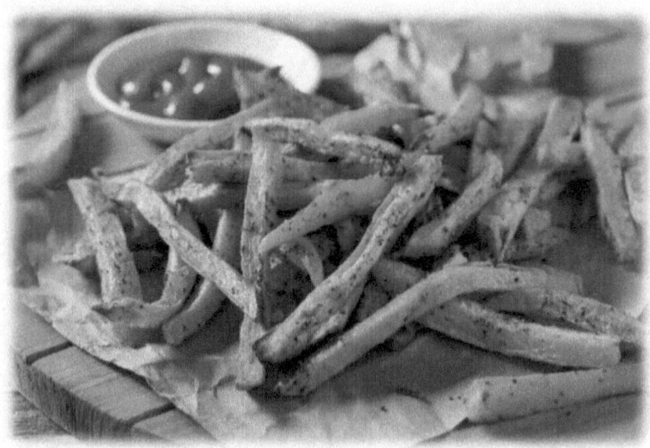

Here the baked sweet potato chips are simply served with lime wedges, but feel free to serve them with your favorite dip: salsa, mayonnaise, guacamole, salsa verde, ...

INGREDIENTS

- 2 medium sweet potatoes, sliced into 1/8- inch thick slices;
- 1 tbsp cooking fat, melted;
- $\frac{1}{2}$ tsp sea salt;
- 1 lime, cut into wedges;

PREPARATION

1 Preheat your oven to 400 F.

2 Coat the sweet potato slices with the melted cooking fat in a bowl and line them on two
bak-
ing sheets, making sure the slices don't touch.

3 Bake them in the preheated oven for 22 to 25 minutes, turning them once, until the edges
are
nice and crisp.

4 Remove the sweet potato chips from the oven and sprinkle them immediately with the sea salt.

5 Serve the chips with lime wedges.